Jean Buttigieg

The Human Genome as Common Heritage of Mankind

STUDIES IN MEDICAL PHILOSOPHY

Edited by Alexander Gungov and Friedrich Luft

ISSN 2367-4377

1   *David Låg Tomasi*
     Medical Philosophy
     A Philosophical Analysis of Patient Self-Perception in Diagnostics and
     Therapy
     ISBN 978-3-8382-0975-3

2   *Jean Buttigieg*
     The Human Genome as Common Heritage of Mankind
     ISBN 978-3-8382-1157-2

Jean Buttigieg

THE HUMAN GENOME AS COMMON HERITAGE OF MANKIND

ibidem-Verlag
Stuttgart

Bibliographic information published by the Deutsche Nationalbibliothek
Die Deutsche Nationalbibliothek lists this publication in the Deutsche Nationalbibliografie;
detailed bibliographic data are available in the Internet at http://dnb.d-nb.de.

Bibliografische Information der Deutschen Nationalbibliothek
Die Deutsche Nationalbibliothek verzeichnet diese Publikation in der Deutschen
Nationalbibliografie; detaillierte bibliografische Daten sind im Internet über http://dnb.d-nb.de
abrufbar.

Cover picture: iStock.com/Lonely__

ISSN: 2367-4377

ISBN-13: 978-3-8382-1157-2

© *ibidem*-Verlag / *ibidem* Press

Stuttgart, Germany 2018

Dedication

I would like to dedicate this thesis to my wife Mariella and my children Emmanuel and Maria Lara in recognition and appreciation of their unwavering support during my studies.

Abstract

There are three main goals that this research study will seek to achieve. The first is to make the human genome, as a common heritage of mankind, a legal principle of international law. Already in 1997, the UNESCO General Conference declared the human genome the common heritage of humanity, in a symbolic sense, in its Declaration on the Human Genome and Human Rights. This declaration was followed by the Joint Statement of 14 March 2000, by President Bill Clinton and British Prime Minister Tony Blair, in which they stated that the 'fundamental data on the human genome, including the human DNA sequence and its variations, should be made freely available to scientists everywhere'. The two leaders' announcement to allow 'unencumbered access' to this fundamental data on the human genome, for the benefit of all humanity, appeared to endorse the UNESCO Declaration of 1997 on the human genome.

But it is our contention that these references to the human genome as common heritage of mankind were only political slogans rather than genuine attempts to make the human genome, as a common heritage of mankind, a legal principle of international law. Our goal is to re-introduce, into public discourse, the philosophical and political implications of the concept of common heritage of mankind, as intended by Arvid Pardo when he addressed the UN General Assembly on November 1, 1967, and apply them to the human genome.

The second goal of this research study is to demonstrate that the biggest challenge to making the human genome the common heritage of mankind comes from the patent system as it is presently operated, that encourages the commercialization of the human genome by denying scientists 'unencumbered access' to the fundamental raw data on the human genome. By putting *individual rights* before *community rights*, the patent system is not conducive to promoting discoveries that improve health by providing new and better medical treatments.

The third goal concerns the issue of biotechnology. While the biotechnology debate is very often centred on what new applications of biotechnology should or should not be permitted, there is missing a critical philosophical analysis of biotechnology itself that can no longer be ignored if we do not want the human genome to fall victim to modern science's project of complete mastery of nature, including human nature. This philosophical analysis should lead to a re-introduction, into public discourse, of the notion that the true essence of the human genome is to be found in metaphysics and not biology. This will entail resisting the trend of modern science to consider as irrelevant any metaphysical considerations on the human genome.

These are the concerns that will be made subject to philosophical scrutiny throughout this research study. In the first chapter, we will be discussing the different ways how the patent system is generating an 'anti-commons' in biomedical research. In the second chapter, we will carry the concept of common heritage of mankind from the deep seabed to the human genome. The metaphysical nature of the human genome will be the subject of the third chapter while in the last chapter we will focus our attention on the contributions of Martin Heidegger and other philosophers on issues concerning technology and biotechnology, in particular. We will also discuss the ways how these philosophical concerns relate to the human genome. The last section will consider a number of political initiatives that can be taken with the purpose of promoting, on the international level, the legal recognition of the human genome as a common heritage of mankind.

Our research study is meant to fill a gap in the literature on the human genome and the common heritage of mankind that tends to ignore the 'anti-commons' effect of the patent system on biomedical research and gives very little importance to the metaphysical nature of the human genome and to the philosophical concerns surrounding the field of biotechnology.

Table of Contents

Acknowledgements

I am deeply indebted to Rev. Professor Emmanuel Agius without whose supervision and intellectual support I would not have been able to conduct this research study.

Introduction
Arvid Pardo and the Human Genome

0.1   The Race to Grab the Bounties
of the Seabed and Ocean Floor

The *nexus* between Arvid Pardo and the human genome is the concept of common heritage of mankind. This concept is synonymous with Pardo who, as Permanent Representative of Malta to the United Nations, presented to the world a revolutionary new idea of international management of the natural resources of our planet Earth that was to challenge the very foundations of economic thinking and international law.[1] He called for the establishment of some form of international management of the seabed and ocean floor that were beyond national jurisdiction.[2] Pardo was concerned that the world's seabeds and much of the ocean floor were subject to exploitation by those countries that had the technology to do so.[3] At the same time, those countries that did not have this technology would end up with nothing. Pardo was personally convinced that the natural resources[4] which were to be found on the seabed and ocean floor were so plentiful that their exploitation by the developing countries could help bridge the gap between the North and the South.[5] This was a golden opportunity for mankind to use the natural resources of the planet in a way that everyone would benefit from them. Pardo's proposal to the United Nations was that all humanity will take it upon itself to create the conditions necessary for the exploitation of the seabed and ocean floor for the benefit of all mankind and set a precedent that would make

---

[1]   Arvid Pardo, Address by Arvid Pardo to the 22nd Session of the General Assembly of the United Nations (1967), Official Records of the General Assembly, Twenty-Second Session, Agenda Item 92, Document A/6695.

[2]   Address by Arvid Pardo to the 22nd Session of the General Assembly of the United Nations (1967), Official Records of the General Assembly, Twenty-Second Session, Agenda Item 92, Document A/6695.

[3]   Jack Barkenbus, *Deep Seabed Resources: Politics and Technology* (New York: Free Press, 1979), p. 33.

[4]   Manganese nodules have been found in all oceans and estimates of their aggregate weight runs into trillions of tons.

[5]   Arvid Pardo, *The Common Heritage of Mankind: Selected Papers on Oceans and World Order 1967–1974* (Malta: Malta University Press 1975), p. 2.

it contingent on mankind to make the preservation of the conditions necessary for the continued existence of humanity, the primary objective of responsibility.[6]

The problem that Pardo faced was that there was no well-defined legal framework that could prevent this unfair exploitation of natural resources because the high seas were still subject to the *laissez faire laissez passer* attitude of Grotius' *Mare Liberum*.[7] He was sure that this ambivalent situation would lead to conflicting claims of appropriation by different countries and inevitably there would be serious tension between the developed countries and the developing ones. He was adamant that the great injustices of the past would not be repeated in the present. In the first lines of his speech, Pardo explained to the General Assembly that:

> The dark oceans were the womb of life; from the protecting oceans life emerged. We still bear in our bodies—in our blood, in the salty bitterness of our tears—the marks of this remote past. Retracting the past, man, the present dominator of the emerged earth, is now returning to the ocean depths. His penetration of the deep could mark the beginning of the end for man and, indeed for life as we know it on this earth. It could also be a unique opportunity to lay solid foundations for a peaceful and increasingly prosperous future for all peoples.[8]

Pardo envisaged a future where the world's seabeds and the ocean floor would be exploited under international auspices for the benefit of the whole of mankind rather than by a few countries for the benefit of the few.[9] For these reasons, Pardo employed the phrase *common heritage of mankind* which implied that no state could appropriate these natural resources because they belonged to all of humanity, those living and also those who still had to be born.[10]

One of the objects of our study will be to show that with the launch of the Human Genome Project (HGP) that marked the beginning of a new era of resource exploitation, that of the human genome, another appeal must be made to

---

[6]   Pardo's proposal is reflected in the Declaration of the Principles Governing the Seabed and the Ocean Floor, and the Subsoil Thereof, beyond the Limits of National Jurisdiction, adopted by the General Assembly of the United Nations at its 25th Session on 17 December 1970.

[7]   Hugo Grotius was a Dutch legal scholar whose 1609 book *Mare Liberum* promoted the idea that seas should be free for innocent use and benefit of all.

[8]   Pardo, *The Common Heritage of Mankind*, p. 2.

[9]   Interim Report on the United Nations and the Issue of Deep Ocean Resources, by United States Congress House Committee on Foreign Affairs Subcommittee on International Organizations, 90th Congress, First Session, 7 December 1967, p. 277.

[10]   Arvid Pardo was not person who coined the term 'common heritage of mankind' because it had already been used by Ambassador A.A. Cocca who was one of the prominent figures in the discussions on the common heritage of mankind and President Lyndon Johnson.

the General Assembly of the United Nations to assume the responsible steward-ship of the human genome through the establishment of some form of interna-tional management as envisaged by Arvid Pardo so as to prevent the unilateral exploitation of the human genome by those nations that have the technical ca-pability to do so. It is also our contention that the situation is more urgent today when the patent system provides the public and private entities that exploit the human genome with proprietary rights that, as we shall demonstrate, have given rise to the *tragedy of the anti-commons*.

Arvid Pardo, in his speech to the General Assembly, specifically avoided referring to these natural resources as belonging to the whole of mankind. What Pardo had in mind and it was in this formulation that he was prophetic, was a new concept of the use of property that was not in any way related to appropri-ation. His was a new vision of resource management where these common re-sources would not be subject to appropriation of any kind, public or private, national or corporate. Sovereignty would be absent as would all legal attributes and ramifications.[11] The notion that the deep sea and ocean resources were the legacy of humanity had already been expressed by President Lyndon Johnson in 1966 but Pardo's idea of common heritage of mankind was diametrically op-posed to that of President Johnson. In 1966, at the inauguration of the *Oceanog-rapher*, Lyndon had said, to the surprise of many:

> Under the circumstances, must we even allow the prospects of rich harvest and mineral wealth to create a new form of colonial competition among the maritime nations. We must be careful to avoid a race to grab and hold the lands under the high seas. We must ensure that the deep seas and the ocean bottom are, and remain, the legacy of all human beings.[12]

President Johnson was very much aware that the race to grab the bounties of the seabed and ocean floor had already started when in 1945 US President Harry Truman declared that the seabed of the continental shelf beneath the high seas but contiguous to the coasts of the US belonged to the US.[13] This action on the part of the Americans prompted other countries to do the same as they too wanted their share of the natural resources to be found on the seabed and ocean

---

[11]   Christopher C. Joynor, 'Legal Implications of the Concept of the Common Heritage of Man-kind', *International and Comparative Law Quarterly*, 35 (1986), 190–199 (p. 191).

[12]   Address given by President Lyndon Johnson at the commissioning of the vessel, *U.S. NOAA Oceanographer*, 13 July 1966.

[13]   Ann L. Hollick, 'US Oceans Policy: The Truman Proclamations', *Virginia Journal of Interna-tional Law*, 17:1 (1976), 23–55.

floor. Proof for the existence of these resources was given in 1873 when the *Challenger* expedition discovered potato-sized manganese nodules scattered across large areas of the seabed at depths of around 3,500 metres.[14] Then in 1958 the Convention of Geneva on the Law of the Sea declared that the coastal states had the sovereign right to exploit and explore the resources of the continental shelf as long as these resources were to be found in depths of 200 metres or less and that they were indeed exploitable.

Pardo was not pleased with this chain of events because he feared that the Geneva Convention could allow a coastal state to divide the seabed and its resources with another coastal state on the opposite side of the sea. In this way, the countries that had the technological means to exploit these resources, and there weren't many countries that had this technology, would have exclusive rights to these undersea resources.[15] The majority of countries, especially the developing ones, lacked this technological capability and they feared that the free exploitation sanctioned by the Geneva Convention would lead to a carve-up of the seabed and all its resources which, according to oceanographers, potentially comprised the largest mineral deposit on this planet.[16] Even though these countries lacked the technology to exploit these resources, they wanted to reserve the right to do so in the future.[17]

Paradoxically, it was an attempt to keep the high seas free for navigation and fair trading that made possible this ambivalent situation where stronger nations could monopolize the high seas for their personal gain and exclude other nations from their share of the prize. The occasion was the seizure, on 25 February 1603, of a richly laden Portuguese galleon by a Dutch Admiral employed by the Dutch East India Company (VOC) in the straits of Malacca as a form of protest against the decision of Spain and Portugal to exclude all foreigners from navigating the Pacific and Indian Oceans. The VOC had only been formed a year before in 1602 and the exclusion policy of Spain and Portugal was preventing it from doing trade with the East.[18] Eager to convince its potential allies of

---

[14]   Barkenbus, *Deep Seabed Resources*, p. 4.

[15]   Pardo, *The Common Heritage of Mankind*, p. 31.

[16]   Barkenbus, *Deep Seabed Resources*, p. 5.

[17]   Ida Ryuichi, 'Human Genome as Common Heritage of Mankind—with a Proposal', *Bioethics in Asia*, 1.8 (1997). <http://www.eubios.info/ASIAE/BIAE59.htm> [accessed on 28 January 2000]

[18]   Jasper A. Bovenberg, *Property Rights in Blood, Genes and Data: Naturally Yours?* (Leiden: Martinus Nijhoff Publishers, 2006), p. 37.

its justification for abducting the Portuguese galleon and the reasons why it took such a drastic form of action, the VOC appointed Hugo Grotius to write a defence in which he would do just this. Grotius was immediately aware that his brief would have very serious implications for the freedom of navigation and more so, for the freedom of trade.[19] As a legal basis for his defence, Grotius turned to natural law as opposed to the man-made laws of a specific nation or jurisdiction. Choosing the Tribunal of Conscience and the Tribunal of Public Opinion as pillars for his defence, he made it clear that the laws of nature written in the minds and hearts of every individual are immutable and universally given.[20] To set the tone for his brief with the serious political and economic implications it carried, Grotius began his defence by stating:

> To this tribunal we bring a new case. It is in very truth no petty case such as private citizens are wont to bring against their neighbours about dripping eaves or party walls; nor is it a case such as nations bring against one another about boundary lines or the possession of a river or an island. No! It is a case which concerns practically the entire expanse of the high sea, the right of navigation, the freedom of trade! Between us and the Spaniards the following points are in dispute: Can the vast, boundless sea be the appendage of one kingdom alone and it not the greatest? Can any one nation have the right to prevent other nations which so desire, from selling to one another, from bartering with one another, actually from communicating with one another? Can any nation give away what it never owned, or discover what already belonged to some one else? [21]

Grotius based his defence for the freedom of the seas and the right to free trade on the distinction, in Roman Law, between two forms of legal ownership, *res nullius* [22] and *res communis*.[23] The question for Grotius was whether the sea was *res nullius* or *res communis*? *Res nullius* referred to those territories and resources that as such belonged to no one by default because no one would have as yet appropriated them or laid claim to them. Legally, however, these territories and resources could be appropriated or exploited by a recognized sovereign

---

[19]   Ibid., pp. 37-38.

[20]   Hugo Grotius, *Freedom of the Seas: The Right of the Dutch to Take Part in the East Indian Trade*, trans. by Ralph Van Deman Magoffin (New York: Oxford University Press, 1916), p. 6. <http://www.oll.libertyfund.org/EBOOKS/Grotius_0049.pdf> [accessed on 22 August 2006]

[21]   Ibid., p. 5.

[22]   Ibid., p. 13.

[23]   Ibid.

if sovereignty or possession could be demonstrated and performed through discovery and effective occupation.[24] Once this process was fulfilled, territories or resources formerly regarded as *res nullius* could become transformed legally into territory subject to the exclusive ownership or jurisdiction of the sovereign who would have started the process in the first place.[25] With *res communis* the situation is totally different because in this case the territories or resources held in common possession could never become appropriated or laid claim to because they had to remain available for use by everyone. Hence these territories were not and could never be subject to sovereign claims of appropriation.[26]

By drawing on this distinction between *res nullius* and *res communis* and how land or resources in the former type of ownership can be subject to appropriation but not in the latter case, Grotius comes to the conclusion that the sea, which as yet had never been the subject of appropriation, was, by default, *res communis* and therefore the claim of Spain and Portugal for exclusive right to the Pacific and Indian Oceans was illegal. His views echoed the position of the second-century Roman Jurist Marcianus, who wrote that the sea, its fish and even coastal waters were *communis omnium naturali jure* and so 'common or open to all men by the operation of natural law'.[27]

However, Grotius did not exclude the possibility that part of the *res communis* can, in actual fact, become subject to private appropriation, as long as the occupation or appropriation is conditional to two fundamental imperatives, namely that the said occupation or appropriation does not impair its *common use* and that if necessity dictates, what is private will become common again. He gives as examples what happens on board a ship when, if food becomes scarce, it is gathered in common, and how the Romans, despite allowing their subjects

---

[24]   *The Institutes of Justinian*, trans. by John Thomas Abdy and Bryan Walker (Cambridge: Cambridge University Press, 1876), pp. 82–85. [Inst. Iust. 2.1.12-18 (De Rerum Divisione)].<http://www.archive.org/details/institutesofjust00abdyuoft> [accessed on 11 April 2004]

[25]   Marjorie M. Whiteman, *Digest of International Law*, 15 vols (Washington D.C.: U.S. Government Printing Office, 1963–1973), II (1963), 1030–1232.

[26]   Pilar N. Ossorio, 'The Human Genome as Common Heritage: Common Sense or Legal', *The Journal of Law, Medicine and Ethics of the American Society of Law, Medicine and Ethics*, 35:3 (2007), 425–39.

[27]   Arvid Pardo, 'The Law of the Sea: Its Past and Its Future', *Oregon Law Review*, 63:1 (1984), 7–17.

to occupy the shoreline, denied them the right to prevent anyone from accessing the shoreline and doing what was traditionally considered permissible.[28]

In conclusion, Grotius makes it clear that Spain and Portugal were wrong in their claim to exclude foreigners from navigating the Pacific and Indian Oceans because the sea was *res communis omnium*,[29] meaning, for the common use of all and so it had to remain. The problem was that as long as the legal framework related to the high seas was primarily concerned with ensuring freedom of navigation and freedom of trade, there was very little concern for disputes between countries related to the use of the high seas. In fact, Grotius' *Mare Liberum* encouraged a *laissez faire, laissez passer* attitude that did not pose any serious international problems for over three centuries after its publication. It was only when the *Challenger*[30] expedition found the manganese nodules on 1873 and US President Harry Truman declared, in 1945, that the US had a claim to the natural resources of the seabed of the continental shelf contiguous to the coasts of the US, that trouble started.[31] Mexico, Panama, Argentina, Peru and many other nations made similar claims for extension of sovereignty over the continental shelf and its resources. The first conflicts involved coastal states and distant-water fishermen over the coastal fish stocks. In 1954, a fishing fleet belonging to the magnate Aristotle Onassis was captured after the Peruvian authorities opened fire on the fleet. The fleet which included a factory ship was flying the Panamanian flag and the incident took place 300 miles off the coast of Peru. A fine of over $3 million had to be paid to have the boats returned.[32]

0.2   The Race to Grab the Bounties of our DNA

The race to grab the bounties of our DNA did not actually start with the launching of the HGP, as many have been led to believe, but rather with the discovery, in 1953, of the molecular structure of DNA by James Watson and Francis Crick.[33] Their discovery set the stage for a new science of the human genome that, with the HGP, has proved to be the gateway to a new biotechnological era.

---

[28]   Bovenberg, *Property Rights in Blood, Genes and Data*, p. 55.

[29]   Abdy, *The Institutes of Justinian*, pp. 78–80.

[30]   Pardo, *The Common Heritage of Mankind*, p. 7.

[31]   Ibid., pp. 18–19.

[32]   Bovenberg, *Property Rights in Blood, Genes and Data*, p. 57.

[33]   James D. Watson, *The Double Helix: A Personal Account of the Discovery of the Structure of DNA* (London: Weidenfield & Nicolson, 1968).

Already Watson and Crick had predicted that their discovery would, in the future, make it possible for scientists to understand biology in terms of physical and chemical processes[34] and even life, for that matter, would be explicable in terms of its molecular structure.[35]

The launching of the HGP by the US National Institutes of Health (NIH) in 1990 promised *oceans of data* as the people behind the HGP set themselves the goal of determining the sequence of the 3 billion chemical base pairs that made up human DNA so as to store the information in a database.[36] The work was completed by April 2003 and the genetic nucleotides were published on the internet along with an estimated 25,000 genes that coded for the proteins that formed our cells and tissues. [37]

But it immediately became clear that these *oceans of data* were susceptible to exploitation[38] because as soon as the multibillion dollar effort to decipher the human genetic code got underway, the Great Gene Grab[39] began! By the time the first draft of the human genome was completed, the map of the human genome was cluttered with flags marking genes that had been patented by biotech companies. If the genome was the moon, then Neil Armstrong would have discovered that large areas of the moon had already been divided among biotech companies before he had the chance to set his foot on it and proclaim, 'one giant leap for mankind'.[40] The irony is that the first hijacker of the human genome was none other than the NIH itself which was among the first to patent the DNA sequence data after two of its scientists discovered a technique that made it pos-

---

[34]   Francis H. C. Crick, *Of Molecules and Men* (New York: Prometheus Books, 2004), p. 19.

[35]   James D. Watson, *The Molecular Biology of the Gene* (New York: W.A. Benjamin, 1965), p. 67.

[36]   Leslie Roberts, R. John Davenport, Elizabeth Pennisi and Eliot Marshall, 'A History of the Human Genome Project', *Science*, 291:5507 (2001), 1195.

[37]   Final HGP papers were published in 2006. A high-quality 'finished' sequence of the human genome was completed in 2003. Involved in the HGP, besides the Department of Energy and the National Institutes of Health, were several researchers at numerous colleges, universities and laboratories throughout the United States that also received funding for human genome research. Many private companies also conducted research that contributed to the success of the HGP.

[38]   Bovenberg, *Property Rights in Blood, Genes and Data*, p. 37.

[39]   Antonio Regalado, 'The Great Gene Grab', *Technology Review* (September/October 2000), 49–50.

[40]   Ibid., p. 49.

sible for them to find genes at an unprecedented speed. Although the NIH eventually withdrew its patent claims, its action triggered a race to the patent office by several countries who also filed patent applications for their own sequences. The UK was the first country to respond, followed by Japan, Germany and Switzerland, all participants to the HGP.[41]

A survey carried out by Kyle Jensen and Fiona Murray focussing on the US has shown that nearly 20% of human genes are explicitly claimed as US Intellectual Property (IP).[42] This figure represents 4382 of the 23,688 of genes in the gene database of the National Centre for Biotechnology Information. These genes that are claimed in 4270 patents within 3050 patent families are owned by 1156 different assignees of which roughly 63% are private firms. Of these, among the top ten we find nine US-based firms, including the University of California, Isis Pharmaceutical, the former Smithkline Beecham and Human Genome Sciences.[43]

While most of the genome is still unpatented, there are some genes that are heavily patented such as BMP7, an osteogenic factor and CDKN2A, a tumour suppressor gene. The gene sequences in both cases are claimed in at least twenty patents, mostly directed towards diagnostic applications. The same holds for other important disease genes such as BRCA1(breast cancer), PIK3R5 (diabetes) and LEPR (obesity).[44]

Many institutions, scientists and individuals are concerned that gene patenting halts scientific progress because it discourages scientists from continuing to do research on genes once they have become patented.[45] Take *Hereditary Hemochromatosis*, for example. It is an autosomal recessive disease affecting mainly people of European descent. Up to 85% of cases of *Hereditary Hemochromatosis* are caused by two mutations in the *Hemochromatosis* gene. While there were several US laboratories performing testing for mutations, as many as

---

[41]   I.J. Demaine and A. X. Fellmeth, 'Reinventing the Double Helix: A Novel and Nonobvious Reconceptualization of the Biotechnology Patent', *Standard Law Review*, 55 (2002), 303–462 (p. 328).

[42]   Kyle Jensen and Fiona Murray, 'Intellectual Property Landscape of the Human Genome', *Science*, 310 (2005), 239–40.

[43]   Ibid.

[44]   Ibid.

[45]   Lori B. Andrews, 'Genes and Patent Policy: Rethinking Intellectual Property Rights', *Nature Reviews*, 3 (2002), 803–08.

30% stopped developing a genetic test or stopped testing for mutations altogether after the gene was patented. As a result, the validation of genetic testing has not proceeded as quickly as it would have if the mutations had not been patented.[46]

The promise and perils of gene patenting can be illustrated with the human epidermal growth factor receptor-2 (HER2) and Tratuzumab (Herceptin). Tratuzumab is an effective antibody against a known breast cancer oncogene which 'instructs' the HER2 gene to either stop the cancer from continuing to spread or to signal to the immune system to destroy the cancer cell. Tratuzumab therapy has been shown to increase survival among women with metastatic as well as localized breast cancer. The downside is that Genetech Inc. which holds the patent for Tratuzumab, also holds multiple patents related to the HER2 gene and HER2 ligands. This means that anyone who wants to develop a breast cancer treatment based on the HER2 gene must obtain permission from Genetech or risk being sued for patent infringement. Hence it is not at all surprising that the drug is so expensive with the annual cost of Tratuzumab therapy in Canada being as high as $50,000.[47]

Professor Emmanuel Agius, Member of the European Group on Ethics (EGE) and others have also expressed their concern as to the patentability and commercialization of genetically engineered living products of biotechnology. Although they have no issue with granting the inventor a just reward for his work, they have expressed serious concerns about the ownership and dominion over living nature, as regulated by the patent system, and are concerned as to how the long-range effects of granting exclusive rights over new life forms can affect the future of the human species.[48] Professor Agius has spoken of the urgent need for a World Patent Convention on Biotechnological Inventions in view of the rapid advances in biotechnology that are being made and in view of the fact that many industrialized countries are increasing their budgets to support the budding biotechnology industry.[49]

---

[46]   Brian Goldman, 'HER2 Testing: The Patent "Genee" Is Out of the Bottle', *Canadian Medical Association Journal*, 176 (2007), 1443–44 (p. 1444).

[47]   Ibid.

[48]   Emmanuel Agius, 'Patenting Life: Our Responsibilities to Present and Future Generations', in *Germ-Line Intervention and our Responsibilities to Future Generations*, ed. by Emmanuel Agius and Salvino Busuttil (Dordrecht: Kluwer Academic Publishers, 1998) pp. 68–69.

[49]   Ibid., pp. 73–74.

The situation faced by Arvid Pardo in 1967 is very similar to the situation that we now face today with the human genome. The human genome consists of genes and genetic information. It is *information* on the life of humanity and accordingly, the human genome should be considered a 'common inheritance'.[50] In addition, as the genes themselves are the place where this genetic information is stored, the genes and genetic information they provide together constitute the common heritage of humanity and as such are *res communis*. Accordingly, the human genome, as *res communis*, cannot be owned by anyone, must be available for use by everyone and can never be appropriated by anyone.[51] It stands to reason that the patent system, based on granting exclusionary rights in the form of intellectual property rights to inventors, is incompatible with declaring the human genome the common heritage of mankind which is a concept based on *community interests* rather than *individual interests*.[52] This will mean striking a balance between rewarding and protecting an inventor for his or her research work and ensuring that inventor's research is made freely and rapidly available to other researchers for the benefit of all mankind.

Arvid Pardo's suggestion to the United Nations General Assembly was to establish some form of international management of the seabed and ocean floor so as to ensure that these resources are explored, prospected and exploited for the benefit of all mankind and so no one is left out. He was faced with the probable monopolization of the resources of the deep seabed by highly developed countries that had the technology to exploit these biological and mineral resources.[53]

---

[50]   On 14 April 2003, in a joint proclamation by six heads of state comprising France, the USA, the UK, Germany and Japan and China, on the 50th anniversary of the discovery of the DNA double helix by James Watson and Francis Crick, it was stated that with the completion of the Human Genome Project, 'all the chapters of the book of human life were complete'.
On 14 March 2000, in a Joint Statement by US President Bill Clinton and UK Prime Minister Tony Blair, it was declared that the 'raw fundamental data on the human genome, including the human DNA sequence and its variations, should be made available to scientists everywhere'.

[51]   Tanya Reimer, *New Property and Global Governance: The Common Heritage of Mankind* (submitted by Tanya Reimer on 24 April 2007 to Dr. O'Brien in partial completion of Global Governance), p. 5. <tanya.peatt.net/published/property_global_gov_chh.pdf> [accessed on 15 May 2007]

[52]   Ryuichi, 'Human Genome as Common Heritage of Mankind', pp. 59–63.

[53]   Pardo, *The Common Heritage of Mankind*, p. 31.

The patenting system as presently practised is mainly centred in the northern hemisphere by developed countries.[54] As it is, the system is contributing in no small measure in widening the gap between the developed and developing countries when multinational firms, owned by the developed countries, are protecting their own interests by acquiring monopoly control through the patent system, over genetic resources and biotechnology.[55] As it is the chances of the Third World to gain access to scientific information and rights to license this technology are being seriously threatened.[56]

A similar situation exists with the human genome because most of the research on the genome is in actual fact monopolized by the highly developed countries. Considering that the objective of research on the human genome is focussed on the improvement of human life and that such research may influence and even decide, the future of each person and so of humanity as a whole, it becomes imperative that the human genome does not remain the object of appropriation by these countries in order to ensure an equitable sharing of the benefits from this common resource among all mankind. Hence, as in the case of the seabed and ocean floor, the current situation calls for some form of international management of the human genome to ensure that the inspiring principles of the concept of common heritage of mankind will not only guarantee the well-being of both the present and future generations of mankind but also thwart any potential threats to mankind by the granting of ownership rights on the human genome.

0.3   The Technology Question

So far our attention on the human genome has focused mainly on making the human genome the common heritage of mankind. This is only the tip of the iceberg because, from a philosophical perspective, our concern must also focus on the subtle way that biotechnology has conditioned the way we look upon the human genome. Biotechnology is a reality that we very easily take for granted because we very often assume that it can only make life better for us as long as we use it within the confines of our legal system. It is our contention that such an approach to biotechnology will only obscure the dangers that are inherent in

---

[54]   Robert Song, *Human Genetics* (Cleveland: The Pilgrim Press, 2002), p. 102.

[55]   Jeremy Rifkin, *The Biotech Century: How Genetic Commerce Will Change the World* (London: Phoenix, 1998), pp. 36–37.

[56]   Agius, 'Patenting Life', p. 69.

the same biotechnology that modern science tends to propose as the key to the solution of all our problems of ill health. It was Martin Heidegger who first subjected technology to philosophical scrutiny with his essay, *The Question Concerning Technology* [57] in which he focused on the way the relation of man to technology has changed as a result of the different manner in which the older forms of technology and modern technology reveal the world to man. At the same time that Heidegger wrote the essay, biotechnology was still a limited application of technology that did not raise any particular ethical concern. The situation is very different today when biotechnology has not only become one of the most powerful technologies in the hands of modern science but it is also considered the technology that poses the most serious threat to mankind![58] For these reasons, the concerns expressed by Heidegger in relation to modern technology are particularly applicable to biotechnology that is the main focus of our study. As we shall make clear in the course of our research, it is only after we have unmasked the dangers inherent in biotechnology that can adversely affect the way we value the human genome will we be able to put the human genome at the centre of biotechnology in the interests of mankind. It is our firm belief that the concept of common heritage of mankind is the most suitable form of resource management of the human genome for and on behalf of all mankind as opposed to the patent system as presently operated that encourages the commercialization of the human genome in the interests of the few.

In his essay, Heidegger begins by describing older forms of technology as a form of *poesis*, which in Greek means to make, to produce and to manufacture and from which the English word for poetry is derived. Viewed in this light, the River Rhine is 'revealed'[59] to man primarily as a source of philosophical inspiration and cultural pride. The same cannot be said of modern technology that stands in a completely different relation to the world which can be best described as one of 'challenging forth' that demands from man an instrumental stance vis-à-vis the world.[60] Using words borrowed from Martin Buber, with modern technology, the 'I and Thou'[61] relation between man and the world is reduced to an

---

[57]   Martin Heidegger, 'The Question Concerning Technology', in *Basic Writings*, ed. by David Farrell Krell (London: Routledge, 1978), p. 318.

[58]   Bill McKibben, *Enough: Staying Human in an Engineered Age* (New York: Henry Holt and Company, 2003), pp. 88–92.

[59]   Heidegger, 'The Question Concerning Technology', p. 321.

[60]   Ibid., p. 320.

[61]   Martin Buber, *I and Thou*, trans. by Ronald Gregor Smith (Edinburgh: T&T Clark, 1999).

'I and It' where the 'It' is man who unknowingly allows himself to be placed in the 'iron cage' of technology![62] In this light, the River Rhine is seen primarily as an energy resource and by the building of a dam, becomes transformed into a hydroelectric power plant. According to Heidegger, this revealing by modern technology of the River Rhine as an 'energy resource', induces an instrumental stance to nature that puts to the River Rhine, the unreasonable demand to supply energy which can be extracted and stored.[63]

The problem for Heidegger is that modern technology does not stop at revealing the world to man as an energy resource but it also reveals man to himself as another energy resource that is challenged forth to be transformed into energy reserve. So, the forester who walks the forest just like his grandfather did in the past, is no longer seen, in an existentialist perspective, as the person who can have a privileged 'I and Thou' relation[64] with nature but, on the contrary, the demands of modern technology make the forester one cog in the machine that puts the paper industry at the mercy of the printing industry that ultimately transforms the public consumer into a source of profit.[65] Seen in this light, the forester is a mere 'It' who must succumb to the demands of modern technology.

For Heidegger, the real threat to man from technology does not come from atomic weaponry or other destructive devices which can destroy us physically. Rather, the threat comes from living under the sway of the technological view of reality that may well destroy the spiritual essence of man.[66] Hence, for Heidegger, the essence of technology is by no means anything technological and therefore it is not to be found in various activities associated with modern technology. Rather, it is to be found in the human impulse to put the world into boxes, to enclose all of our experiences of the world within categories of understanding that we can control.[67] This impulse to control the world which Heidegger calls 'enframing' is the essence of technology and as such it precedes and determines the development of modern science.[68]

---

[62]   Charles Taylor, *The Ethics of Authenticity* (Cambridge M.A.: Harvard University Press, 1991), pp. 93–108.

[63]   Heidegger, 'The Question Concerning Technology', p. 321.

[64]   Buber, *I and Thou*, pp. 19–21.

[65]   Heidegger, *Basic Writings*, 'The Question Concerning Technology', pp. 323–24.

[66]   Michael E. Zimmerman, 'Beyond "Humanism": Heidegger's Understanding of Technology', in *Heidegger the Man and the Thinker*, ed. by Thomas Sheehan (Chicago: Precedent Publishing, 1981), p. 224.

[67]   Mahon O'Brien, *Commentary on Heidegger's 'The Question Concerning Technology'*, in IWM Junior Visiting Fellows' Conferences, Vol. XVI/I, 2004.

[68]   Heidegger, *Basic Writings*, pp. 325–26.

However, Heidegger is not content with merely identifying 'enframing' as the essence of modern technology—he proceeds to demonstrate how human beings should stand in relation to technology. For Heidegger, the question about how we are to relate to technology always comes too late since we are already caught up in an 'enframing' view of nature as much as we are caught up in the concrete realities of technological development. Nonetheless, he believes that we can gain some perspective on our own orientation to the world and in so doing, achieve a perspective on technology. What is crucial to Heidegger is that we establish a free relationship with both the world and modern technology because it is the same impulse that has attracted man towards understanding the world and the process of revealing that rules in modern technology. There is a *continuum* between the way the River Rhine is today revealed as an energy resource and the manner in which a silver chalice was, in the past, revealed by the silversmith's handiwork which brought it out of concealment. Prior to the silversmith's work on the raw material from which the chalice was made, the chalice was only potentially a chalice and this potentiality became actualized in the hands of the silversmith and so the chalice is revealed.[69]

For Heidegger, that which poses the threat also contains the possibility of rescue within itself. He believes that we can achieve a balanced life and keep technology in its place.[70] This means entering into a new relation with technology which will involve being able to walk away from it in order to free ourselves from it so as to become aware of the transcendent dimension within which we exist.[71] Inspired by the work of Heidegger, Charles Taylor argues, in his *Ethics of Authenticity*, that although we may appear to live in an 'iron cage',[72] still we remain free to remake the conditions of our existence when we choose to dominate the things that tend to dominate us. Accordingly, instead of seeing technology in the context of an ever-increasing control and domination, he argues in favour of working towards an alternative 'enframing' of technology understood in the moral frame of an ethics of practical benevolence.[73]

---

[69]   Ibid., pp. 313–16.
[70]   Richard Polt, *Heidegger* (London: Routledge, 1999), p. 174.
[71]   Zimmerman, 'Beyond "Humanism"', p. 226.
[72]   Taylor, *Ethics of Authenticity*, pp. 93–108.
[73]   Ibid., p. 101.

In a slightly more negative vein, Hans Jonas acknowledges that human ingenuity has engendered a giant mechanism and no one can tell what its ultimate repercussions may be:

> Outstanding in prestige and starving in resources whatever belongs to the fullness of man, the expansion of his power is accompanied by contraction of his self-conception and being.[74]

Still, like Heidegger, he believes that the 'remembrance of Being' should become a spur to the ethical betterment of humanity in the here and now.[75] Although we cannot remove the technological threat we have brought about, just as we cannot do away with technology itself as it is indispensable for our survival, the prevention of its disastrous consequences must represent a constant task for moral theory.[76] Hans Jonas was one of the first philosophers to speak about the inadequacy of traditional ethical theories in relation to the extension of human power through the advancement of technology and the need to take action to counteract this power. [77] For Jonas, with the advent of modern technology, man's power to change the world for the better or for the worse increased to such an extent that the adequacy of pre-technology ethical thinking began to be called into question. Prior to the advent of modern technology, the effective range of human action was relatively localized, and as such, nature was immune from any serious harm resulting from man's actions.[78] But with the power that *homo faber* [79] was able to harness from nature, the consequences of man's actions became entirely unpredictable.

Today, while man is very much aware of the power he has to change himself through biotechnological intervention and the biosphere through technological intervention, he is very little aware of how he himself is being shaped in ways that he cannot comprehend by the same technology that he thinks he has under his complete control. The *Imperative of Responsibility* is Jonas' answer to

---

[74]   Hans Jonas, *The Imperative of Responsibility: In Search of an Ethics for the Technological Age* (Chicago: University of Chicago Press, 1984), p. 23.

[75]   Richard Wolin, *Heidegger's Children* (Princetown: Princetown University Press, 2001), p. 119.

[76]   Hans Jonas, 'Wissenschaft as Personal Experience', *Hastings Center Report*, 32:4 (2002), 27–35 (p. 34).

[77]   Jonas, *The Imperative of Responsibility*, p. 6.

[78]   Hans Jonas, *Philosophical Essays: From Ancient Creed to Technological Man* (Chicago: Chicago University Press, 1974), p. 6.

[79]   Ibid., p. 10.

the 'heuristics of fear' [80] that must guard mankind against the unpredictable consequences of ever more powerful technologies that today include nuclear technology, robotics and biotechnology among others:

> [Man ought] not to ruin (as he well can do) what nature has achieved in him by the way of his using it. Beyond this commitment to himself, he becomes the custodian of every other end in itself that ever falls under the rule of his power.[81]

Arvid Pardo and Hans Jonas have taken it upon themselves to carry out this moral task to warn the world community about the disastrous effects that technology can have on the future of mankind. Both Pardo and Jonas had their own different stance towards technology unlike Heidegger who preferred to escape away from technology by choosing to go and live in the Black Forest for the later period of his life.[82] At one end of the spectrum, Jonas adopted an extremely cautionary stand in relation to technology for fear of letting instrumental reason, the product of the technological age, to subjugate mankind to a process of dehumanization that will ultimately deprive us of our humanness. At the other end of the spectrum, Pardo had no qualms about the positive contribution technology could make to human society. His sole concern was that technological capability would not be used as a tool in the hands of the developed countries to deprive the less-developed and technologically advanced countries from benefiting from the resources of the deep seabed as they lacked the technology to do so. It is for this reason that he chose to propose to make the deep seabed the common heritage of mankind.

Many today are showing the same concerns expressed by Pardo and Jonas when they see the human genome becoming more patentable subject matter and less common heritage of mankind with every day that passes. On the one hand, the patenting system, based on free-market thinking, does not ensure an equitable sharing in the benefits that are accrued from the exploitation of the data acquired from studies on the human genome. On the other hand, the threat of dehumanization posed by technology to the human species has assumed a new

---

[80]   Jonas, *The Imperative of Responsibility*, pp. 26–27.
[81]   Ibid., pp. 129–30.
[82]   Beginning in the summer of 1922, Heidegger occupied a small, three-roomed cabin overlooking the small mountain town of Todtnauberg, in the Black Forest.

dimension with a biotechnology that can be used to make alterations to the human genome![83]

The public was understandably overwhelmingly enthusiastic about the benefits that would result from the data collected by the HGP researchers when the full sequence of the last chromosome was published in the magazine *Nature*[84] in May 2006. Everyone was anxious to see how this vast storehouse of genomic information could be rapidly developed into new products to diagnose and treat human disease. Many recalled the words of US President Bill Clinton who had announced on 26 June 2000, after the completion of a 'working draft' DNA sequence of the human genome, that the data offered mankind the possibility to learn the language in which God created man and that the knowledge acquired from this data would give mankind an immense power to heal.[85] Three months earlier, on 14 March 2000, Bill Clinton and Tony Blair had stated that the 'raw fundamental data on the human genome, including the human DNA sequence and its variations, should be made freely available to scientists everywhere'.[86]

But scientists who are trying to understand human biology and disease at the level of individual genes with the aim of providing better diagnostics, treatments and cures have in fact been denied 'unencumbered access'[87] to this fundamental data because of the exclusive proprietary rights that the patent system grants to patentees. The truth of the matter is that the patent system is proving to be an obstacle to the promotion of health and the prevention of disease.

Scientists will not be able to proceed effectively with their research if they are not given the freedom to choose their own research objectives and method. For Michael Polanyi, the most effective way of organizing scientific research is by having independent initiatives undertaken by competing scientists. In this way, as long as a scientist keeps an eye on the work of other scientists, he will

---

[83]   Leon R. Kass, *Life, Liberty and the Defence of Dignity: The Challenge for Bioethics* (San Francisco: Encounter Books, 2002), pp. 219–39.

[84]   S. Gregory and others, 'The DNA Sequence and Biological Annotation of Chromosome', *Nature*, 441: 7091 (18 May 2006), pp. 315–321.

[85]   On 26 June 2000, President Bill Clinton at the White House and Tony Blair at 10 Downing Street simultaneously proclaimed the first draft of the Human Genome Project complete. <http://www.ornl.gov/hgmis> [accessed on 20 March 2006]

[86]   Bill Clinton and Tony Blair, Joint Statement by President William Clinton and Prime Minister Tony Blair of the United Kingdom (14 March 2000) <http://wwwipmall.info/hosted_resources/ippresdocs/ippd_44.htm, 14 March> [accessed on 20 March 2006]

[87]   Ibid.

take their efforts into account when formulating his own research questions. Polanyi has labelled this system as a 'system of self-coordination by way of mutual adjustments of independent initiatives'.[88] This coordination should not be centralized but rather it should be guided by an 'invisible hand' similar to the 'invisible hand' of a free market economy that encourages producers and consumers to make supply meet demand and thus achieve maximum welfare.[89] Likewise, the 'invisible hand' of research will guide scientists to achieve maximum progress of science.[90] This method of doing science can be guaranteed by making the human genome the common heritage of mankind which is a concept based on *community interests* rather than *individual interests*.[91]

In the following chapters, we will demonstrate how a 'common heritage' model of management of the human genome, inspired by Arvid Pardo's prophetic vision of resource management, will ensure an equitable sharing of the benefits that can be derived from research on the human genome. Despite the fact that a number of contemporary authors have shown a renewed interest in the concept of common heritage of mankind, they have failed to analyse the concept from a philosophical perspective. This explains the difficulties that international lawyers and economists encounter when they try to make sense of the conundrum of meanings that have been attributed to the common heritage of mankind. In our study we will consider the common heritage of mankind as first and foremost a philosophical concept that has its roots in natural law and the model of Good Stewardship. The advantage of this approach is that we will be able to demonstrate the original meaning that Arvid Pardo intended to give the concept of common heritage of mankind and then apply this to the human genome.

We will also propose the creation of a model of governance of the human genome on the same lines as the International Seabed Authority that will be referred to as the International Human Genome Authority. This Authority will be able to provide an ethical foundation for all biotechnological inventions and discoveries that are derived from the human genome. In order to achieve this, the establishment of the Authority must be accompanied by (i) a re-thinking of the patent system and (ii) a re-evaluation of the biotechnology debate that tends to

---

[88]   Michael Polanyi, 'The Republic of Science: Its Political and Economic Theory', *Minerva*, I (1962), 54–74.

[89]   Taylor, *Ethics of Authenticity*, pp. 93–107.

[90]   Polanyi, 'The Republic of Science', pp. 54–74.

[91]   Ryuichi, 'Human Genome as Common Heritage of Mankind', pp. 59–63.

obscure the relevance of metaphysical considerations on the human genome. In the next section of our study, we will be focussing our attention on issues related to the patentability of the human genome and 'anti-commons' effect that the patenting system has on biomedical research. We will also discuss the reasons why the human genome was declared to be the 'common heritage of humanity, in a symbolic sense' and the reasons why we consider the patent system that grants exclusive property rights to inventors, to be incompatible with the concept of common heritage of mankind.

Chapter One
The Human Genome—Common or Patentable Subject Matter?

1.1   The Human Genome as Common Heritage

While the application of the patent system in the field of biotechnology and biomedicine has seemed justifiable in the past as a way of ensuring a reasonable
balance between the rights of inventors and the public interest, the granting of
patents that assert rights over DNA sequences have raised special concern
among individuals, scientists, national and international organizations. Most of
these concerns have revolved around the idea that human DNA is of a special
nature compared to the DNA of other organisms. Many are troubled by the idea
that genes and their mutations can be subject to commercialization. Others are
very concerned about the fact that the patent system in the field of biotechnology
is in actual fact an impediment to the progress of scientific research with tragic
consequences for healthcare.[92] These same concerns have encouraged many to
try to encourage the adoption of new legislation that would guarantee a more
equitable and sustainable use of biotechnology. These concerted efforts have
produced a number of notable results, including the Council of Europe Convention on Biomedicine[93] with its related Protocol on Human Cloning,[94] the Universal Declaration on the Human Genome and Human Rights[95] with the related

---

[92]   Nuffield Council of Bioethics, *The Ethics of Patenting DNA: A Discussion Paper* (London:
       Nuffield Council on Bioethics, 2002), pp. 21–22.
[93]   Council of Europe Convention for the Protection of Human Rights and Dignity of the Human
       Being with Regard to the Application of Biology and Medicine: Convention on Human Rights
       and Medicine, Oviedo, 4 April 1997, CETS 164.
[94]   Council of Europe Additional Protocol to the Convention for the Protection of Human Rights
       and Dignity of the Human Being with Regard to the Application of Biology and Medicine, on
       the Prohibition of Cloning Human Beings, Paris, 12 January 1998, CETS 168.
[95]   Universal Declaration on the Human Genome and Human Rights, adopted by the General Con-
       ference of UNESCO at its 29th Session on 11 March 1997.

Declaration on Human Genetic Data,[96] and the Declaration on Human Cloning.[97] The Council of Europe's Committee on Legal and Human Rights has also called on member states to change the basis of patent law with respect to rights of ownership over human tissue and genes into 'law pertaining to the common heritage of mankind'.[98]

Expressing the same concerns and taking into account the fact that the EU Directive on the Legal Protection of Biotechnological Inventions[99] was being challenged at the European Court of Justice by the governments of the Netherlands and Italy and that Norway was inclined not to implement it,[100] the Parliamentary Assembly of the European Union found it expedient to recommend that member states should strive towards establishing a 'World Patent Convention' which would replace the present patent system that is considered to be inadequate for dealing with the discovery of human genes in particular.[101] The Parliamentary Assembly also recommended that this proposed system should be founded on a principle of common heritage of mankind which should reflect the language of the Universal Declaration on the Human Genome and Human Rights.[102]

The Universal Declaration on the Human Genome and Human Rights was adopted unanimously and by acclamation by the General Conference of UNESCO on 11 November 1997, as a result of the urgent need felt by the international community to provide itself with an international instrument more particularly focussed on the human genome.[103] While the concept of common her-

---

[96]   International Declaration on Human Genetic Data, adopted by the General Conference of UNESCO at its 32nd Session on 16 October 2003.

[97]   Declaration on Human Cloning, adopted by the General Assembly of the United Nations at its 59th Session on 8 March 2005. UNGA Resolution 59/280.

[98]   Parliamentary Assembly of the Council of Europe Recommendation 1512 (2001) on the Protection of the Human Genome.

[99]   Directive 98/44/EC of the European Parliament and of the Council of 6 July 1998 on the Legal Protection of Biotechnological Inventions. OJL 213, 30 July 1998, pp. 13–21.

[100]   Parliamentary Assembly of the Council of Europe Recommendation 1425 (1999) on Biotechnology and Intellectual Property, para. 8.

[101]   Ibid.

[102]   Parliamentary Assembly of the Council of Europe Recommendation 1468 (2000) on Biotechnologies.

[103]   With Resolution 29C/17, entitled 'Implementation of the Universal Declaration on the Human Genome and Human Rights', the General Conference of UNESCO laid out the methods for the implementation of the Declaration.

itage of mankind had gradually spread throughout the international law, particularly in the 1960s with the law of the sea, this was the first time that the concept was extended to the specific nature of humankind itself.[104]

On 9 December 1998, the Declaration was endorsed by the United Nations General Assembly.[105] The Preamble of the Declaration recalls the aims and principles of the Declaration which are fully in line with the ideals of UNESCO and the ethical mission it assigned itself in its constitution. In the field of human genetics, this mission inevitably becomes acute with regards to the risks incurred by humankind, such as the risk of calling into question the principle of the equal dignity of persons, the risk of an erosion of the social and moral solidarity of societies towards vulnerable persons and the risk of the growth of inequalities in the sharing of benefits from research and its applications. The Declaration affirms the intrinsic value that is attached to preserving the unity of the human race by stating in Article 1 that,

> The human genome underlies the fundamental unity of all members of the human family, as well as the recognition of their inherent dignity and diversity. In a symbolic sense, it is the heritage of humanity.[106]

This proclamation is considered the cornerstone of the Declaration.[107] According to the Committee of Governmental Experts, all subsequent provisions of the Declaration proceed from the innovative nature of this proclamation.[108] When applying the term 'common heritage of humanity' to the human genome, the Declaration made it clear that genetic research should engage the responsibility

---

[104]   'Fourth Meeting of the Legal Commission of the IBC' (Paris, 27 April 1994), in *Birth of the Universal Declaration of the Human Genome and Human Rights* (UNESCO: Division of the Ethics of Science and Technology, 1999), pp. 53–54.

[105]   Resolution 53/152 on The Human Genome and Human Rights, adopted by the United Nations General Assembly at its 53rd Session on 9 December 1998.

[106]   Universal Declaration on the Human Genome and Human Rights, adopted by the General Conference of UNESCO at its 29th Session on 11 March 1997.

[107]   'Eight Meeting of the Legal Commission of the International Bioethics Committee' (Paris, 16–17 December 1996), in *Birth of the Universal Declaration of the Human Genome and Human Rights* (Paris: UNESCO, 1999), p. 107; 'Revised Preliminary Draft of a Universal Declaration on the Human Genome and Human Rights' (20 December 1996), in *Birth of the Universal Declaration of the Human Genome and Human Rights* (Paris: UNESCO, 1999) pp. 153–56.

[108]   'Revised Preliminary Draft of a Universal Declaration on the Human Genome and Human Rights' (20 December 1996), in *Birth of the Universal Declaration of the Human Genome and Human Rights* (Paris: UNESCO, 1999) pp. 153–56.

of the whole of humanity and, more importantly, that the results of this research should benefit all of humankind, present and future generations.[109] Article 1 of the Declaration stresses the deep interrelatedness, from a genetic perspective, that should exist between all members of the human species, by asserting that human genes are common to all past, present and future generations as the same genetic structure is inherited from one generation to the next, and therefore, each individual should inherit the same basic genetic structure of those that preceded him or her.[110]

Article 1 of the Declaration also proclaims the human genome, 'in a symbolic sense, the heritage of humanity'.[111] The justification for including the human genome in the common heritage of mankind is based on the characteristics it shares with commons such as the seabed and the moon. This formula was successfully applied to marine space in the framework of the Conference on the Law of the Sea,[112] and the moon in the framework of the Moon Treaty.[113] Nevertheless, the formula does not really fit a reality such as the human genome which, unlike marine space and the moon, represents both a general dimension inasmuch as it is an element common to the whole of the human species and an individual dimension inasmuch as it is the distinctive element of every human being who receives it from his/her parents in the act of conception. Hence the notion of the human genome refers both to the full set of genes of each individual, comprising both genetic material and genetic information, and to the entire range of genes which constitute the human race. For this reason the drafters of the Declaration used the term 'genome' in a metonymic sense in order to incorporate the twin senses of the human genome. So, by using the term 'symbolic sense', the drafters were referring to (a) the human genome (part) which was representative of (b) the common features of the human genome (whole) which constituted the common heritage of mankind.

---

[109] Hector Gros Espiell, *Genese de la Declaration Universelle sur le Genome Humain et les Droits de l'Homme* (Paris: UNESCO, 1999), p. 3.

[110] Agius, 'Patenting Life', p. 76.

[111] Declaration on Human Genome, Article 1.

[112] United Nations Convention on the Law of the Sea (UNCLOS), Montego Bay, 10 December 1982.

[113] 1979 Agreement Governing the Activities of States on the Moon and Other Celestial Bodies, adopted by the General Assembly of the United Nations at its 34th Session on 5 December 1979. UNGA Resolution 34/68.

In stating that the human genome is, symbolically the heritage of mankind, Article 1 affirmed the fundamental unity of the human species and the value of preserving it by stressing the inter-relatedness of the human family, the common genetic blueprint and the shared future of mankind. This notion is intended to convey the idea that the human genome engages a responsibility from and for all of humanity and, (i) is not suitable for appropriation by any state or private entity; (ii) requires a management system in which all users have rights and benefits are shared and (iii) is reserved for peaceful purposes and preserved for future generations.[114]

Still, there are some writers who have argued that if the human genome is considered the basis of the dignity and unity which characterize the whole human species, then such a proposal could be interpreted as implying a purely reductionist biological definition of the human genome.[115] It was specifically in order to pre-empt such a possibility, that the drafters of Article 1 preferred to use the phrase 'in a symbolic sense [the human genome] is the heritage of humanity', [116] instead of the original one proposed by the International Bioethics Committee (IBC) which began the first article with a categorical and at the same time, ambiguous statement, 'the human genome is the common heritage of humanity'.[117] The IBC wording was dropped in favour of the modified version because of fears that it might be used to dilute individual rights in favour of eugenic policies.[118] Roberto Andorno comments on the same lines when he says that Article 1 may be interpreted in such a way that the eminent value attached to the human person is solely based on the genetic information that characterized our species—this interpretation would be contrary to the intention of the drafters as it clearly results from other provisions of the Declaration, especially Article 2[119]

---

[114]   Pardo, *The Common Heritage of Mankind*, pp. 40–41.
[115]   Giorgio Filibeck, 'Protecting Human Genome is the Responsibility of all Humanity: Observations on the Human Genome Declaration Recently Adopted by the General Conference of UNESCO', *L'Osservatore Romano*, 11 February 1998, p. 10.
[116]   Hector Gros Espiell, 'Introduction', in *Birth of the Universal Declaration on the Human Genome and Human Rights* by UNESCO (Paris: UNESCO, 1999), p. 3.
[117]   UNESCO, *Birth of Universal Declaration*, pp. 121–56.
[118]   Ryuichi, 'Human Genome as Common Heritage of Mankind'. [accessed on 28 January 2000]
[119]   Declaration on Human Genome, Article 2.

and Article 6[120] which stress that people cannot be reduced to their genetic make up.[121]

What is surprising is that while the principle of the common heritage of mankind precludes the appropriation of common space areas and recommends that any benefit derived from such areas should be distributed among the whole of mankind, the Declaration fails to address or condemn gene patenting which grants exclusive property rights to inventors. By putting individual rights before community rights, the patent system is widely criticized as being an obstacle to not only the development and progress of medicine and genetics but also to the protection of human rights.[122] According to these critics of the patent system, the human genome must remain free from commercialization which will only happen when scientific research is no longer impeded by exclusive intellectual property rights. Only then will all of mankind, including people from the least developed countries, be able to share in the benefits derived from human genome research, including economic benefits.[123]

According to the Chairman of the Legal Commission, Hector Gros Espiell, the human genome falls under the purview of both civil law and international law. It came under civil law with its responsibilities since it constituted the distinctive element specific to each individual as a component of his or her uniqueness and could be transmitted as heritage. At the same time the human genome came under international law in virtue of being the common heritage of humanity as it was part of the common gene pool of the human species as a whole, which transcends individual genetic identities.[124] In this context, it must be rec-

---

[120] Ibid., Article 6.

[121] Roberto Andorno, 'Human Dignity and the UNESCO Declaration on the Human Genome', in *Ethics, Law and Society*, ed. by Jennifer Gunning and Soren Holm (Aldershot: Ashgate, 2005), pp. 73–84.

[122] 'The Significance of UNESCO's Universal Declaration on the Human Genome and Human Rights' (2005) 2:1 SCRIPT-ed 18-47. <http://www.law.ed.ac.uk/ahrb/script-ed/vol2-1/harm on.pdf> [accessed on 30 May 2006]

[123] UN Sub-Commission on the Promotion and Protection of Human Rights, *Specific Human Issues: Working Paper on Universal Declaration on the Human Genome and Human Rights*, submitted by Antoanella-Iulia Motoc, 15 August 2002, E/CN.4/Sub.2/2002/37. <http://www.u nhcr.ch/Huridocda/Huridoca.nsf/0/91ea34c7ea607bb4c1256c1a0058857c/$FILE/GO215047. doc> [accessed on 10 May 2007]

[124] UNESCO, *Birth of Universal Declaration*, p. 47.

orded that the term 'common heritage of mankind' was used in Article 1, paragraph 3 of the Declaration of the Principles of International Cultural Co-operation:

> In their rich variety and diversity, and in the reciprocal influences they exert on one another, all cultures form part of the common heritage of mankind.[125]

According to Gros Espiell, the fact that in this Declaration on World Cultures, it is categorically stated that all cultures form part of the common heritage of mankind, then it can be logically inferred that every single human being is the depository of both his or her own genome and the genome of the entire species. It follows, argues Espiell, that every member of the human species must consider himself or herself the custodian of not only his or her own personal genome but also the genome of the entire species that must remain the expression of the richness and diversity of all cultures that form the common heritage of mankind.[126]

Gros Espiell also commented that although the concept of common heritage of humanity had gradually spread throughout international law—in particular in the early 1960s in the Law of the Sea—this was the first time it was extended to the specific nature of humankind itself, which is at the same time the most personal part of a human being, namely the genome.[127] Hence, to the Chairman of the Legal Commission, the term 'humanity' was a legally applicable concept and therefore the subject of international law, with rights and responsibilities towards itself and towards future generations.[128]

It was decided, during the consultation process, to insert in the Declaration the principle of the non-patentability of the genome. But the drafters refused to do so for a number of reasons:

---

[125] Declaration of the Principles of International Cultural Co-operation, proclaimed by the General Conference of UNESCO at its 14th Session on 4 November 1966.

[126] Hector Gros Espiell, 'Project of an International Instrument for the Protection of the Human Genome' (12 September 1994), in *Birth of the Universal Declaration on the Human Genome and Human Rights* (Paris: UNESCO, 1999), pp. 41–48.

[127] 'Fourth Meeting of the Legal Commission of the IBC' (Paris, 27 April 1994), in *Birth of the Universal Declaration of the Human Genome and Human Rights* (Paris: UNESCO, 1999), pp. 53–54.

[128] Ibid.

1) Classifying the human genome as part of the common heritage of humanity was to serve as a reminder that knowledge about the human genome can never be the privilege of the few but must benefit humanity as a whole—this helped ensure free access to research data on the human genome;[129] the ethical imperative that the human body and its elements and products are part of the heritage would theoretically proscribe the patentability of human genes.[130]

2) The principle of free access was not incompatible with patenting the results of genome research—free access to such results was deemed to be guaranteed while respecting intellectual property rights.[131]

However, in terms of the classic distinction in patent law between inventions which could be patented and discoveries which could not, it remained unclear whether the results of human genetic research could be patented.

The distinction between inventions and discoveries remains one of the principle concerns in the controversial debate about the ownership rights that the patent system awards the patentee. Many are of the opinion that as genes are naturally occurring entities, they can only be discovered and not invented.[132] On the other hand, there are others who are of the opinion that once a gene is isolated from the human body, it becomes a patentable invention. In fact, the drafters' response to the claim that the non-patentability of the human genome be recognized was that isolating and defining a protein-coding gene was not, in fact, a mere discovery but a patentable invention. The basic problem was to determine how, in that area, to best serve the interests of humanity as a whole.[133]

From a legal point of view, it was argued that it would be very difficult to assert that classifying the human genome as the common heritage of humanity would automatically exclude any possibility of patenting genome research. Nor could patenting be excluded entirely when it could serve to stimulate genome research on which future therapeutic progress depended. The drafters eventually

---

[129] Hector Gros Espiell, 'Mechanism for Monitoring the Future Universal Declaration on the Human Genome and Human Rights' (1 July 1996), in *Birth of the Universal Declaration on the Human Genome and Human Rights* by UNESCO (Paris: UNESCO, 1999), Observation 4, p. 70.

[130] Ibid.

[131] Ibid.

[132] Nuffield Council, *The Ethics of Patenting DNA*, pp. 22–23.

[133] UNESCO, *Birth of Universal Declaration*, p. 70.

refused to define the precise purpose of declaring the human genome to be common heritage subject matter.[134]

This refusal to proclaim the non-patentability of the human genome contrasted with the Declaration's affirmation of the principle of solidarity, on a practical level, as expressed by the concept of common heritage. The Declaration, in fact, proclaims that

a) Benefits from advances in biology, genetics and medicine, concerning the human genome, shall be made available to all, with due regard for the dignity and human rights of each individual.

b) Freedom of research, which is necessary for the purpose of knowledge, is part of freedom of thought. The applications of research, including applications in biology, genetics and medicine, concerning the human genome, shall seek to offer relief from suffering and improve the health of individuals and humankind as a whole.[135]

The problem is that while the Declaration acknowledges the right to pursue research, necessary for the progress of knowledge and freedom of thought as a human right, its concept of solidarity is more linked to states/groups and individual duties rather than rights. With respect to states, the Declaration proclaims that they should foster conditions favourable for ethical research, ensure that research is not used for non-peaceful purposes and recognize the value of establishing multi-disciplinary ethics committees independent from political, economic, scientific and medical authorities.[136] Accordingly, states should ensure solidarity towards genetically vulnerable individuals, families and populations by fostering research on the identification, prevention and treatment of genetically-based and influenced diseases, both rare and endemic. There should also be scientific and cultural co-operation between developed and developing states through the dissemination of scientific knowledge 'concerning the human genome, human diversity and genetic research'.[137] This expression of solidarity and international co-operation will help towards preventing the gap between the developed and developing states from continuing to widen. Finally, in the same spirit of international solidarity, states should encourage measures that will enable developing states to benefit from scientific and technological research.[138]

---

[134] Bovenberg, *Property Rights in Blood, Genes and Data*, p. 45.
[135] Declaration on Human Genome, Article 12.
[136] Ibid., Articles 14, 15 and 16.
[137] Ibid., Article 18.
[138] Ibid., Article 19.

But as such the Declaration does not offer any guidance as to how these practical applications of international solidarity could be achieved. More importantly, from a legal point of view, the drafters' refusal to recognize that patentability was irreconcilable with the notion of the human genome as common heritage meant that it would be very difficult to assert that classifying the human genome as the common heritage of humanity automatically excluded any possibility of patenting genome research.[139]

The Declaration was more direct in its application of the principle of solidarity with respect to individuals with Article 10 stipulating that human rights must take precedence over research.[140] Article 12 also stipulates that the benefits from advances in biology, genetics and medicine concerning the human genome should be made available to all and that the research carried out should be directed to the improvement of health and relief from suffering.[141] Article 13[142] identifies the ethical duties incumbent on every researcher while Articles 11[143] and 24[144] prohibit research contrary to human dignity such as human reproductive cloning and germ-line interventions.

It is unfortunate that while the Declaration has provided against the exploitation of the human genome, in its natural state, for financial gains, it has left open the question as to whether the human genome can be patented for research purposes?[145] This has been a primary concern for many scientists, national and international organizations and individuals since the Declaration was adopted in 1997. The issue has acquired greater significance in view of the fact that in the field of genetics, it has become increasingly difficult to establish a clear distinguishing line between inventions that may be patented and discoveries that may not.[146]

---

[139]   UNESCO, *Birth of Universal Declaration*, p. 70.

[140]   Declaration on Human Genome, Article 10.

[141]   Ibid., Article 12.

[142]   Ibid., Article 13.

[143]   Ibid., Article 11.

[144]   Ibid., Article 24.

[145]   Aurora Plomer and others, *Stem Cell Patents: European Patent Law and Ethics*, European Commission (28 July 2006). <http://www.nottingham.ac.uk/law/StemCellProject/project.reports.htm> [accessed on 12 June 2007]

[146]   Rebecca Eisenberg, Re-Examining the Role of Patents in Appropriating the Value of DNA Sequences, *Emory Law Journal*, 49 (2000), 783–800.

1.2 The Human Genome as Patentable Subject Matter

A serious obstacle to the implementation of the provisions of the UNESCO Declaration is the EU Database Directive of 1996 which conferred a strong and potentially exclusive property right in the collection of data and information. This Directive converted data and information which were previously the unprotectable raw materials of the modern information economy into the subject matter of a new exclusive property right that is paradoxically more powerful in certain key aspects than a patent. The novel right to protection for database producers created by the EU Database Directive has seriously undermined all efforts to consider the human genome as the common heritage of mankind.[147] While the Declaration leaves open the issue of the patentability of the human genome, the Directive gives database producers a *sui generis* right of protection without requiring them to account for the patentability of their databases. At the same time, this protection creates new and potentially serious obstacles to biomedical research owing to the multiplicity of new owners of upstream information who are granted exclusive property rights and so can impose heavy fees for researchers to make use of their database.[148] The result of such a situation is the creation of an anti-commons,[149] where a proliferation of intellectual property rights leads paradoxically to fewer useful products for improving human health.

Originally, the primary objective of the Directive was to provide builders of databases with adequate legal protection to ensure them a just return on their investment in building their databases. The issue became more pressing when it became evident that while databases were expensive to create, they could be copied very cheaply.

Accordingly, the EU Directive was meant to achieve two primary goals, namely to harmonize the domestic laws of the different EU member states in respect of databases by adopting a single intellectual creation standard for copyright protection and to ensure the protection of the contents of databases. With

---

[147] Directive 96/9/EC of the European Parliament and of the Council of 11 March 1996 on the Legal Protection of Databases. OJL 77, 27 March 1996, pp. 20–28.

[148] J.H. Reichman, 'Saving the Patent Law from Itself: Informal Remarks Concerning the Systemic Problems Afflicting Developed Intellectual Property Regimes', in *Perspectives on Properties of the Human Genome Project*, ed. by F. Scott Kieff (Amsterdam: Elsevier Academic Press, 2003), pp. 297–99.

[149] Michael A. Heller and Rebecca S. Eisenberg, 'Can Patents Deter Innovation? The Anticommons in Biomedical Research', *Science*, 280 (1998), 698–701.

regards to the first goal, the EU Directive sought to define what constituted a database in terms of its selection or arrangement of material such that it could be considered the personal intellectual creation of its maker.[150] The second objective, on the other hand, sought to protect the contents of the database.[151]

But in the process, the Directive created a controversial *sui generis* right[152] aimed at protecting the investment of a database builder without setting reasonable conditions for determining the characteristics that must be present for a collection of genetic data to be considered as a database and to qualify for this added protection. The Directive provides that,

> In accordance with this Directive, databases which, by reason of the selection or arrangement of their contents, constitute the author's own intellectual creation shall be protected as such by copyright. No other criteria shall be applied to determine their eligibility for that protection.[153]

Then in Article 7 (1) the Directive sets out to establish the criteria that should determine whether the maker of a database qualifies for the *sui generis* right of protection that the Directive provides. Here the Directive demonstrates a lack of coherence in that while in Article 3 (1) it leaves open the question of what actually should constitute a 'database', in Article 7(1) it indiscriminately gives added protection to practically any builder of a database who has invested substantially in his creation.

> Member states shall provide for a right for the maker of a database which shows that there has been qualitatively and/or quantitatively a substantial investment in either the obtaining, verification or presentation of the contents to prevent extraction and/or re-utilization of the whole or a substantial part, evaluated qualitatively and/or quantitatively, of the contents of that database.[154]

The anomaly is that for a database right to attach, the database builder does not have to bother with the patent concerns of the European Patent Convention (EPC) which include: (i) the criteria for determining what constitutes patentable

---

[150]   Directive 96/9/EC, Article 1.
[151]   Ibid., Articles 2–6.
[152]   Ibid., Articles 7–11.
[153]   Ibid., Article 3 (1).
[154]   Ibid., Article 7 (1)

subject matter; [155] (ii) the exceptions to patentability and the issue of *ordre public*;[156] and (iii) the statutory requirements of novelty,[157] inventive step [158] and industrial application.[159]

The problem is that though genetic databases qualify for the protection provided by the Directive, the Directive itself was not designed with this type of database in mind. It is also questionable whether the DNA sequence databases that are being built today by private and public sector genomics companies, *prima facie* qualify as the kind of database the Directive had in mind when it was published in 1996. Many are concerned by the present situation whereby any database can qualify as valuable intellectual property with the right to supplementary legal protection as long as it is subject to the conditions set forth in the Directive and in full compliance with the limits imposed by the EU member states. To complicate things further, the Directive does not specify whether the database right should be conferred to the builder of the database at large, such as a consortium, for example, or to the individual contributors to the database, keeping in mind that the nucleotide bases are built from the contributions of numerous compilations of partial sequences. In other words, do these compilations or records qualify as databases in their own right and if so, can their contributors claim a database right with respect to their contribution?[160]

The primary concern remains, however, that the Database Directive has marked a radical shift from the historical limits of intellectual property in the past. While traditionally the very concept of public domain was preserved by the proviso that with regards to intangible creations, only temporary exclusive rights were granted, the EU Database Directive confers to the database builder a new exclusive property right in perpetuity with no concomitant obligation to pass on to the public domain the ownership of protection after a specified period.[161]

---

[155] European Patent Convention (EPC 1973), Article 52. <http://www.epo.org/patents/law/legal-texts/html/epc/1973/e/ma1.html> [accessed on 12 June 2007]

[156] Ibid., Article 53.

[157] Ibid., Article 54.

[158] Ibid., Article 56.

[159] Ibid., Article 57.

[160] Bovenberg, *Property Rights in Blood, Genes and Data*, pp. 76–81.

[161] J.H. Reichman and Paul F. Uhlir, Promoting Public Good Uses of Scientific Data: A Contractually Reconstructed Commons for Science and Innovation (A Working Paper in progress). <http://www.law.duke.edu/pd/papers/reichmananduhlir.pdf> [accessed on 10 March 2008]

The Database Directive also marked a fundamental difference from other prerequisites of patent protection.[162] As such the database right is attached to any maker or builder of a database in which collection, verification or presentation of its contents demonstrated quantitatively or qualitatively a substantial investment and automatically the maker/builder of the database was exempt from the criteria for patentability as applied, for example, by the United States Patent and Trademark Office (USPTO)[163] or the European Patent Office (EPO).[164]

1.3   The Anti-Commons of Biomedical Research

The main rationale of the patenting system is that it promotes scientific progress and technological development by providing incentives for inventors, investors and entrepreneurs. When a patent is granted, an inventor is given a right of ownership of his/her invention for a specified period after which the right of ownership is passed onto the public. In exchange for the protection given, the inventor must disclose information about his/her invention with the patent application. For the USPTO, for example, a patent application is normally judged on four criteria, namely, (i) utility; (ii) novelty; (iii) non-obviousness and (iv) enablement. In general, raw products of DNA are not patentable but they become patentable when they have been isolated, purified or modified to produce a unique form not found in nature. Currently over 3 million genome-related patent applications have been filed. Patent applications are confidential until a patent is issued and so determining which sequences are the subject of patent applications is impossible.

For genetic patents, inventors must identify a novel genetic sequence, specify the sequence's product, specify how the product functions in nature and enable one skilled in the field to use the sequence for its stated purpose. Patents have been issued on genes, gene fragments, single nucleotide polymorphisms (SNPs),[165] gene tests, proteins and stem cells.

---

[162]   Reichman, 'Saving the Patent Law from Itself', pp. 297–99.

[163]   United States Patent and Trademark Office. <http://www.uspto.gov/> [accessed on 12 June 2007]

[164]   European Patent Office <http://www.epo/org> [accessed on 12 June 2007]

[165]   SNPs are DNA sequence variations that occur when a single nucleotide in the genome sequence is altered. Many SNPs have no effect on cell function but scientists believe that others could predispose people to disease or influence their response to a drug. This makes SNPs of great value for biomedical research and for developing pharmaceutical products or medical diagnostics.

The patenting of gene fragments is controversial because the effort to find any given expressed sequence tag (EST) is small compared with the work of isolating and characterizing a gene and gene product, finding out what it does, and developing a commercial product. Holders of gatekeeper-patents exercise excessive control over the commercial fruits of genome research. Similarly, allowing multiple patents on different parts of the same genome sequence, such as on a gene fragment, a gene or a protein, adds undue costs to the researcher who wants to examine the sequence. The researcher not only wants to pay each patent holder via licensing for the opportunity to study the sequence but he also has to pay off his own staff to research different patents and determine which are applicable to the area of the genome he/she wants to study. These are the causes that give rise to the anti-commons[166] in the biotechnology industry. As a result, researchers are impeded from making new discoveries and developing new products. Several comments to this effect were sent by the public to the USPTO when it revised its policy guidelines to be used by office personnel in their review of patent applications. These were some of the comments:

i.   While inventions are patentable, discoveries are not and genes are discoveries rather than inventions.[167]

ii. Patents should not be issued for genes because patents on genes are delaying medical research and thus there is no societal benefit associated with gene patents.[168]

iii. The scope of patent claims directed to DNA should be limited to applications or methods of using DNA and should not be allowed to encompass the DNA itself.[169]

iv. DNA patent claim scope should be limited to uses that are disclosed in the patent application because allowing patent claims that encompass DNA itself would enable the inventor to assert claims to speculative

---

[166] David B. Resnik, 'A Biotechnology Patent Pool: An Idea Whose Time Has Come?', *The Journal of Philosophy, Science and Law*, 3 (2003). <http://www6.miami.edu/ethics/jpsl/archives/papers/biotechPatent.html> [accessed on 5 February 2005]

[167] United States Patent and Trademark Office (2001), Utility Examination Guidelines', Federal Register, vol. 66. no. 4, pp. 1092–93, Comment 1. <http://www.uspto.gov/web/offices/com/sol/notices/utilexmguide.pdf> [accessed on 14 March 2005]

[168] Ibid., p. 1094, Comment 7.

[169] Ibid., pp. 1094–95, Comment 10.

uses of the DNA that were not foreseen at the time the patent application was filed.[170]

v.   DNA should be freely available for research.[171]

vi. DNA sequences should be considered unpatentable because sequencing DNA has become so routine that determining the sequence of a DNA molecule is not inventive.[172]

Other comments stated that as genes were constituent elements of the human genome that was considered to be the common heritage of mankind then they should not be patented as this would give proprietary rights to the patentees. But the USPTO vehemently rejected this general objection to the issuing of patents on genes arguing that:

> The patent system promotes progress by securing a complete disclosure of an invention to the public, in exchange for the inventor's legal right to exclude other people from making, using, offering for sale, selling or importing the composition for a limited time.[173]

The publication of the Revised Guidelines by the USPTO was a missed opportunity for the US government to put an end to the *tragedy of the anti-commons* in the area of biomedical research, a situation which, ironically, the patent system is supposed to avoid!

1.4   Patenting Life

A significant page in the history of patenting in the US was written in 1980 when the Supreme Court of the United States ruled that a living micro-organism was patentable matter under the provisions of patent laws enacted by Congress in 1952. In 1972, Ananda Chakrabarty,[174] a microbiologist, had filed a patent application assigned to General Electric Company, asserting multiple claims re-

---

[170]   Ibid., p. 1095, Comment 11.

[171]   Ibid., Comment 12.

[172]   Ibid., Comment 13.

[173]   United States Patent and Trademark Office (1999), 'Revised Interim Utility Examination Guidelines', Federal Register, vol. 64 no. 244. <http://www.uspto.gov/web/offices/com/sol/notices/utilexmguide.pdf> [accessed on 18 April 2005]

[174]   Daniel J. Kevles, *A History of Patenting Life in the United States with Comparative Attention to Europe and Canada: A Report to the European Group on Ethics in Science and Technologies* (Luxembourg: Office for Official Publications of the European Communities, 2002), pp. 14–39.

lated to a novel bacterial strain that he had obtained with the aid of genetic engineering. Chakrabarty's bacterial strain could degrade many components of crude oil and so was potentially useful in the biological control of oil spills. Chakrabarty claimed patent rights for the method of producing the bacteria, for the method of carrying the bacteria to water-borne oil spills and for the bacteria themselves. The last claim, initially rejected by the patent examiner and the Patent Office Board of Appeals, was eventually granted on appeal by the United States Court of Customs and Patents Appeals (CCPA) in 1979, which decision was affirmed by a narrow five-four vote of the Supreme Court a year later. [175] The five-four majority vote in this case was partly determined by the role that another company, the Upjohn Pharmaceutical Company played when it withdrew its patent application for a purified version of an antibiotic-producing strain of streptomycin invented by Dr Malcolm E. Bergy[176] that appeared in nature but was in an unpurified state.[177]

Both applications were initially denied by the USPTO because they involved living things but the CCPA, predecessor of the present Court of Appeals for the Federal Circuit, ruled three to two that the patents should be granted, as nothing in patent law barred the issuing of a patent to an otherwise patentable invention simply because it was alive.

The USPTO appealed the Bergy and Chakrabarty patent claims to the Supreme Court but the claims were sent back to the CCPA for reconsideration on the basis of the Supreme Court's ruling on mathematical algorithms in *Parker* v. *Flook*.[178] However, the CCPA again reiterated that as biological conversions mediated by micro-organisms were basically an application of chemistry, there was no reason for not granting the patents for Bergy and Chakrabarty simply because the antibiotic strain of Bergy or the petroleum-eating enzyme of Chakrabarty were alive.

---

[175] U.S. Supreme Court – *Diamond v Chakrabarty*, 447 U.S. 303 (1980), argued on 17 March 1980 and decided on 16 June 1980.

[176] The United States Court of Customs and Patent Appeals, Application of Bergy 596 F. 2d 952 (1979).

[177] Gerald J. Mossinghoff, 'The Evolution of Gene Patents Viewed from the United States Patent Office', in *Perspectives on Properties of the Human Genome Project*, ed. by F. Scott Kieff (Amsterdam: Elsevier Academic Press, 2003), pp. 14–15.

[178] U.S. Supreme Court – *Parker* v. *Flook*, 437 U.S. 584 (1978), argued on 25 April 1978 and decided on 22 June 1978. <http://www.supreme.justia.com/us/437/584/case.html> [accessed on 14 August 2007]

This second opinion was again appealed to the Supreme Court by the USPTO. However, in the meantime, the Upjohn Pharmaceutical Company which owned the Bergy application decided to withdraw its product claims covering its streptomycin which produced the antibiotic lyncomycin on the advice of their lawyers that the Supreme Court would be reluctant to grant a patent for a modified living micro-organism that occurred in nature, even though in a less purified state. This move paved the way for the Supreme Court to grant the Chakrabarty patent claim with a majority of five to four as it found that the creation of a new form of bacteria was a human invention even though it involved living matter.[179] Unlike the Bergy streptomycin, the Chakrabarty enzyme did not occur in nature and so the Supreme Court was less hesitant to grant the patent in these circumstances.[180] In giving its decision, the Supreme Court declared that 'anything under the sun made by man' was patentable and with this broad approach to the patenting of living systems, the USPTO abandoned its long-standing practice of not granting patents for live organisms and began granting patents for micro-organisms and other biotechnological inventions.[181]

From a philosophical perspective, the 'patenting of life' decision of the Court is disturbing for a number of reasons. Judges are not supposed to make the law but only interpret it—it is up to legislative bodies to make the law. In the Chakrabarty case, the statements made by the judges are alarming because they decisively reduce life to the level of matter. Their position is a reflection of the complete certainty that exists among essentially all biochemists that the characteristics of living organisms can be completely understood in terms of the co-ordinative interactions of large and small molecules.[182] This opinion, echoed in numerous scientific essays, is exemplified by Richard Dawkins in his celebrated book, *The Blind Watchmaker*.[183] It is the opinion expressed by Judge Giles Rich when, speaking on behalf of the majority, he contended that micro-organisms were 'much more akin to inanimate chemical compositions such as reactants,

---

[179]   Karen Lebacqz, 'Who "Owns" Cells and Tissues?', *Health Care Analysis*, 9:3 (2001), 356–68 (p. 355).

[180]   Mossinghoff, 'The Evolution of Gene Patents Viewed from the United States Patent Office', p. 13.

[181]   Matthew Rimmer, *Intellectual Property and Biotechnology: Biological Inventions* (Cheltenham: Edward Elgar publishing, 2008), p. 26.

[182]   Watson, *The Molecular Biology of the Gene*, p. 67.

[183]   Richard Dawkins, *The Blind Watchmaker: Why the Evidence of Evolution Reveals a Universe Without Design,* 2nd edn (New York: W.W. Norton & Company, 1996), p. 112.

reagents, and catalysts than they are to horses and honeybees or raspberries and roses'.[184] It is also the opinion of Judge Howard T. Markey, who commented that, 'no congressional intent to limit patents to dead inventions lurks in the lacuna of the statute, and there is no grave or compelling circumstance requiring us to find it there'.[185] Again, when the CCPA ruled in favour of granting the patent after the Supreme Court sent the appeal back to the CCPA for re-consideration, the CCPA ruled in favour of granting the patent, emphasizing that, 'no legally significant difference between active chemicals which are classified as dead and organisms used for their chemical reactions which take place because they are alive'.[186]

An *amicus* brief,[187] sent to the government by the Peoples' Business Commission, argued that to patent life was not in the public interest and the 'issuance of a patent on a life form was to imply that life has no vital or sacred property and it was simply an arrangement of chemicals or composition of matter'.[188] Many are concerned that the deliberations of the judges which made the patenting/ownership of life forms a reality were based on dubious scientific speculation mainly inspired by the scientific approach to life of Erin Schrödinger, who argued that life could be thought of in terms of the storing and transmission of biological information.[189] According to Schrödinger, so much information had to be packed into every cell that it had to be compressed into what he called a 'hereditary code-script' embedded in the molecular fabric of chromosomes. So, in order to understand life, including human life, all one had to do was identify these molecules and crack their code.[190] As the entire complex of living things is based on chains of the same four DNA compounds with each organism having its own distinctive sequence of them, the genetic code is the same for all living

---

[184] Kevles, *History of Patenting Life*, pp. 19–20.
[185] Ibid., p. 20.
[186] Ibid., p. 28.
[187] Several amicus briefs were filed by many individuals and organizations to support or oppose the case after the Solicitor General petitioned the Supreme Court for a ruling. These amicus briefs are documents that are filed in court by individuals and groups who are not directly linked to the case in court but feel that with the information they have in their possession they can assist the court in deciding on the matter at hand.
[188] A. M. Chakrabarty, 'Patenting Life Forms: Yesterday, Today and Tomorrow', in *Perspectives on Properties of the Human Genome Project* (Amsterdam: Elsevier Academic Press, 2003), pp. 4–5.
[189] Erwin Schrödinger, *What is Life?* (Cambridge: Cambridge University Press, 2007), pp. 19–31.
[190] James D. Watson, *DNA: The Secret of Life* (New York: Alfred A. Knopf, 2003), pp. 35–36.

organisms from bacteria to humans with a basic constitutive mechanism that is common to all living organisms. It is this apparent uniformity of the workings of the genetic code in all living things that has induced scientists to think of biological organisms in terms of their physical and chemical mechanisms. To this effect, Francis Crick had claimed that, 'the ultimate aim of the modern movement in biology is in fact to explain all biology in terms of physics and chemistry'.[191] However, he was later to admit that science was not able to explain 'how an organism constructs a hand with its thumb and four fingers, with all the bones, the muscle, and the nerve cells assembled and correctly connected together'.[192]

Crick's last observation unmasks the complexity of the process involved in the generation of new life behind the apparent simplicity of the chemical composition of the DNA molecule.[193] Completely chemical and physical explanations for certain crucial aspects of living things have not been found in spite of the momentous discovery of the molecular structure of DNA. It has generally been assumed that since organisms are essentially living mechanisms and since all mechanisms, be they biological or non-biological, work in accordance with physical and chemical laws, then the same laws must apply to living organisms. According to Michael Polanyi, such explanations of living things can never be found:

> This is not to deny that there is a great deal of truth in the mechanical explanation of life. The organs of the body work much like machines, and they are subject to a hierarchy of controls, exercised by an ascending series of mechanical principles. Biologists pursuing the aim of explaining living functions in terms of machines have achieved astounding success. But this must not obscure the fact that these advances only add to the features of life which cannot be represented in terms of laws manifested in the realm of inanimate nature.[194]

There are two aspects of a mechanism that must be taken into account. There is (i) the factual aspect which comprises the physical and chemical conditions that permit the physical and chemical reactions specific to the particular mechanism taking place and (ii) the boundary aspect that sets conditions or limits within

---

[191]   Crick, *Of Molecules and Men*, p. 10.
[192]   Duncan Ronald and Weston-Smith Miranda, *The Encyclopaedia of Ignorance: Everything You Ever Wanted To Know About the Unknown* (New York: Pocket Books, 1978).
[193]   Michael Polanyi and Harry Prosch, *Meaning* (Chicago: University of Chicago Press, 1975), p. 165.
[194]   Michael Polanyi, *The Tacit Dimension* (New York: Doubleday & Company, 1967), p. 42.

which the particular physical and chemical reactions take place. It is these boundary conditions that determine the pattern in which the physical and chemical interactions are put together in one way rather than in another.[195] When we think of organisms only in terms of physical and chemical reactions, we are only taking into account the physico-chemical principle of the organism. In so doing, we are ignoring the crucial fact that a mechanism acquires its organization by reference to some aim or goal or purpose that is to be achieved by it and this purpose cannot be deduced from the physico-chemical aspect alone.[196]

The USPTO does not allow patents on products of nature or on scientific formulae.[197] But it allows patents on human genes. As a matter of fact, patents on human genes straddle the boundary between patentable and unpatentable substances because DNA sequences are not simply molecules—they are also information. This means that patent claims to *information* represent a fundamental departure from the traditional patent bargain. Originally, the patent-bargain allowed a patent on an invention in exchange for the disclosure of useful information in the application to spur on other inventors.[198] When Judge Rich, speaking on behalf of the majority of the CCPA ruled in favour of the Bergy and Chakrabarty patent claims, he emphasized that the *Parker* v. *Flook* case that rejected patent claims on mathematical algorithms had no bearing whatsoever on these two cases.[199] The CCPA viewed Bergy's strain of streptomycin and Chakrabarty's petroleum-eating enzyme as merely products of human ingenuity and so patentable. Following the Supreme Court's decision on the Chakrabarty case, the USPTO began to accept claims for the patenting of living things both if they were genetically modified as Dr Chakrabarty's enzyme or if isolated and

[195]   Marjorie Grene, 'Reducibility: Another Side Issue?', in *Interpretations of Life and Mind: Essays Around the Problem of Reduction*, ed. by Marjorie Grene (London: Routledge and K. Paul, 1971), p. 18.

[196]   Michael Polanyi, 'Life Transcending Physics and Chemistry', *Chemical and Engineering News*, 45 (21 August 1967), 54–66.

[197]   USPTO, 2106 Patent Subject Matter Eligibility [R-6] 2100 Patentability (26 October 2005). <http://www.gov/web/offices/pac/mpep/docu,ments/2100_2106 htm> [accessed on 18 April 2006]

[198]   Rebecca Eisenberg, 'How Can You Patent Genes?', in *Who Owns Life?,* ed. by David Magnus, Arthur Caplan and Glenn McGee (New York: Prometheus Books, 2002), pp. 117–34.

[199]   U.S. Supreme Court – *Parker* v. *Flook*, 437 U.S. 584 (1978), argued on 25 April 1978 and decided on 22 June 1978. <http://www.supreme.justia.com/us/437/584/case.html> [accessed on 14 August 2007]

purified by the 'hand of man' as Dr Bergy's streptomycin.[200] As was expected, once patents were granted for living organisms, then it was not long before the USPTO began granting patents on human genes and DNA segments.[201]

Many institutions, scientists and individuals consider the USPTO's decision to patent human genes as a fundamental mistake for several reasons. While the fundamental objection remains that of creating a commodity from a part of the human body, the more pressing concern is whether human genes meet the criteria for patentability and so can be considered to be patentable subject matter. In the first place, the useful properties of a gene's sequence are not properties that scientists invent but rather natural inherent properties of the genes themselves. Secondly, gene patents do not meet the criteria of non-obviousness because with today's technology, the functions of human genes can be predicted on the basis of their haemology to other genes. Thirdly, human nucleotide sequences should not be patented, as a matter of public policy, even if their function is known because they represent a kind of scientific knowledge which should remain available to all.[202] The fact that a patent holder has a monopoly over his patent from the date of the patent creates serious problems for public health and biomedical research. The effects on diagnosis and treatment are such that various policy options such as litigation, legislative, patent pools and compulsory licensing are being explored so as to ensure that patents do not impede the practice of medicine and scientific progress. As patent law now stands, a patent holder can control any use of his/her gene by preventing a doctor from testing a patient's blood for a specific gene mutation that is covered by the patent. The patent holder can also prevent others from duplicating the patent holder's research evaluating it. Gene patent holders have prevented some researchers from searching for cures for genetic diseases as happened with wild-type BRCA1 and BRCA2 genes.[203] A researcher who wishes to find a cure for breast cancer must negotiate with not only the patent holders for these two genes but also with all the other patent holders who have discovered and patented any of the hundreds of mutations in these genes.

---

[200] Mossinghoff, 'The Evolution of Gene Patents Viewed from the United States Patent Office', p. 15.

[201] Lebacqz, 'Who "Owns" Cells and Tissues?', p. 356.

[202] Andrews, 'Genes and Patent Policy', pp. 803–08.

[203] Roger Tatoud, *Genes and Ownership: A Scientific Approach* (London: openDemocracy Ltd, 2002). <http://www.openDemocracy.net/theme_9_genes/articles_767.jsp> [accessed on 10 January 2005]

According to common heritage arguments, genes are a kind of public property or *res communis* that belongs to no one person.[204] Genes are considered analogous to other resources common to all people such as public land, the oceans and the atmosphere and so as to protect and preserve this common heritage, specific norms of legal control such as patenting should not be allowed. Critics of common heritage arguments assert that genes are not like natural resources because they cannot be equated with particular objects, processes or locations since the human genome is an abstraction rather than a concrete thing, more akin to a map or schematic diagram than to a piece of tissue, plant or animal. They argue that while the Planet Earth is a natural resource, the map of the Planet is not and so there is no basis for considering the human genome as part of our common heritage.[205]

Since the US Supreme Court ruled in 1980 that life-forms could be patented if they were the products of human ingenuity, the USPTO has awarded patents on plants, animals, cells, organs, proteins and genes. In assessing patent applications, the USPTO has followed the Chakrabarty standard in deciding what counts as patentable subject matter. But what has the Chakrabarty decision achieved? According to Leon Kass, at least one important lesson, if we are willing to learn from it, of how close we have come in our thinking, if not in our practice, to overstep the sensible limits of the project for the mastery and possession of nature. To him this project can only make sense if we fully understand and accept the limited meanings of mastery and possession and only if we appreciate the nature of living nature and our place within it. On these deep matters, the Court, for Kass, was a teacher of shallowness.[206] In its eagerness to serve innovation, the Court, maybe unwittingly, became the teacher of scientific reductionism when it contended that micro-organisms were 'akin to inanimate chemical compositions'.[207]

Paradoxically, while the USPTO has granted patents on plants, animals and genes, those who argue against the idea that genes could be part of the common

[204] David B. Resnik, *Owning the Genome: A Moral Analysis of DNA Patenting* (New York: State University of New York Press, 2004), p. 77.

[205] A. Serano Merlo, 'The Meaning of Genome in Living beings: a Biophilosophical Approach', in *Human Genome, Human Person and the Society of the Future*, ed. by J. de Dios Vial Correa and E. Sgreccia (Vatican City: Libreria Editrice Vaticana, 1999), p. 471.

[206] Leon R. Kass, *Towards a More Natural Science: Biology and Human Affairs* (New York: The Free Press, 1985), p. 149.

[207] Kevles, *History of Patenting Life*, pp. 19–20.

heritage consider the human genome as a map or an abstraction rather than as a tissue, plant or animal!

From a biophilosophical point of view, the patenting of human genes in isolation as if they existed as separate entities outside a larger whole which is none other than the human genome is mistaken. Human genes are the constitutive elements of the human genome and function only within the dynamics of the human genome. The human genome can refer to both the quantitative and qualitative totality of human genes. Quantitatively it can refer to those parts of the DNA in a single individual that are the carriers of the genetic programme that is unique in every single human being and which essentially directs our development as an organism. Qualitatively the human genome can refer to the genetic programme which comprises both the genetic instructions in the DNA of each cell and the organic living structure in which the genetic programme is operative. This second sense of the human genome corresponds to Aristotle's *entelechy* and is the basis not only for the inalienable dignity of each human being but also the basis for a universal moral obligation towards any human being and his genome irrespective of whether he or she is conscious and healthy or not.[208] This is the same sense of the human genome that was used in the Declaration of Principles of International Culture Cooperation which used the notion of common heritage of mankind in the context of the diversity of the world's cultures.[209] According to this formula, each human being is considered to be the depository both of his or her genome and of the genome of the entire species. Viewed in this perspective, the human genome creates responsibilities towards oneself and specific obligations with the object of protecting the genetic diversity of humanity.

The human genome does not comprise only the genetic instructions which are unique to each one of us. Even if the human genome were the genetic information contained in the single genes, the adding up of the information contained in these genes does not make the human genome just as a collection of bricks does not make a house or a collection of car parts does not make a car. Nonetheless, it is the 'information model' that has defined the theoretical framework

---

[208]   Aristotle, *Physics*, trans. by Robin Waterfield (Oxford: Oxford University Press, 1999), 3.1.200b, 12–201b, 29, pp. 56–62.

[209]   Declaration of the Principles of International Cultural Co-operation, proclaimed by the General Conference of UNESCO at its 14th Session on 4 November 1966, Article 1(3).

for the empirical results of genetic research.[210] Notwithstanding, from a biophilosophical perspective, the information content of the human genome is nothing less than the living being as a whole in a strictly teleological sense. From this follows that the human genome must be understood as a genuine whole comprising a unique genetic programme that can be read and actualized only in the living organism and therefore requires the mysterious and irreducible reality of human life to achieve any of its effectiveness. Hence the ontological being, nature and dignity of the human person are grounded in the essential nature of the human person which cannot be changed by manipulating the human genome.[211]

Regrettably the USPTO has chosen to consider human genes as primarily chemical compounds which qualify as compositions of matter with respect to patent criteria. Patents have been granted for particular DNA sequences, whole transcribed genes as complementary DNA (cDNAs), individual mutations, expressed sequence tags (ESTs) and single nucleotide polymorphisms (SNPs). The USPTO also allows process patents which comprise processes, methods or techniques based on identifying, cloning, isolating, modifying, recombining or sequencing genes. The underlying thinking behind the USPTO's policy of granting these genetic patents is Erin Schrödinger's description of the structural and thermodynamic properties of living cells in terms of the storage and transmission of genetic information. To this effect, Schrödinger had written:

> Chromosomes…contain in some kind of codified script, the entire pattern of the individual's future development and of his functioning in the mature state. Every complete set of chromosomes contains the full code.[212]

The problem with Schrödinger's explanation of the molecules of living cells is that it fails to explain the mystery and depth of human life. As things stand, the legal system behind the granting of patents on the chemical structure and function of DNA sequences rejects the notion that genes cannot be reduced to DNA sequences or that their functional properties cannot be entirely explained by their chemical composition.

---

[210] Merlo, 'The Meaning of Genome in Living beings', p. 471.

[211] J. Seifert, 'Respect for Nature and Responsibility of the Person', in *Human Genome, Human Person and the Society of the Future*, ed. by J. de Dios Vial Correa and E. Sgreccia (Vatican City: Libreria Editrice Vaticana, 1999), pp. 363–64.

[212] Schrödinger, *What is Life?*, p. 21.

1.5   Biotechnological Patents versus Public Morality

The EPC uses as a supplementary means of interpretation the Directive on the Legal Protection of Biotechnological Inventions. [213] However, unlike the USPTO, the European Patent Office (EPO) has included a morality clause in its criteria for patentability and it can exclude from patentability any invention that may threaten public morality or *ordre public.* On the basis of this morality clause, European patents are not granted in respect of biotechnological inventions which include processes for the cloning of human beings, processes for modifying the germ line genetic identity of human beings and uses of human embryos for industrial or commercial purposes as they are considered to be contrary to public morality.[214] Processes for modifying the genetic identity of animals which are likely to cause them suffering without any substantial medical benefit to man or animal are also not patentable as are animals that may result from such processes.[215]

The human body at the various stages of its formation and development is also not patentable as is the simple discovery of one of its elements, including the sequence or partial sequence of a gene. However, when an element is isolated from the human body or is produced by means of a technical process, including the sequence or partial sequence of a gene, then such an element may constitute a patentable invention even if the structure of the element is identical to that of its natural element.[216]

Biotechnological inventions are also patentable if they concern biological material[217] that has been isolated from its natural environment or produced by means of a technical process even though the biological material already exists in the natural state.[218]

The morality clause of the EPO proved itself effective when, in 1999, after it granted a patent to the University of Edinburgh on a method of using genetic engineering to isolate stem cells, including embryonic stem cells, the patent was

---

[213]   Directive 98/44/EC of 6 July 1998.

[214]   Ibid.

[215]   European Patent Convention Article 53(a).

[216]   European Patent Convention, Rule 23a.

[217]   'Biological material' includes any material containing genetic information and capable of reproducing itself or being reproduced in a biological system.

[218]   EPC, Rule 23c.

challenged and subsequently amended.[219] The challenge was successful because the patent was considered contrary to the EPC which excludes the patentability of processes that use human embryos for industrial purposes or commercial uses and inventions contrary to *ordre public.*[220]

The fact that the EPC has included a morality clause that has proved effective in prohibiting embryonic stem cell patents shows that it is possible to implement regulation that will benefit the population at large. Another strong stand was taken by the EPO in 2004 when its Examining Division refused a patent by the Wisconsin Alumni Research Foundation for cell cultures comprising primate embryonic stem cells that used pre-implantation embryos as the primary source for generating embryonic stem cell lines capable of remaining stable, undifferentiated and pluripotent for at least one year.[221] A similar stand was taken by the Canadian Supreme Court when it turned down a patent application by Harvard University on a genetically modified mouse that is highly susceptible to cancer, despite the fact that the patent was granted in the US, Japan and Europe.[222]

After ten years of tense and controversial debates, the European Union (EU) adopted the Directive 98/44/EC of the European Parliament and the Council of Europe on the Legal Protection of Biotechnological Inventions on 6 July 1998.[223] In the context of EU legislation, this Directive was the first legal instrument specifically dealing with bioethics. The very long debate involved in the adoption of the Directive was mainly due to conflicts between the economic interests and ethical values at stake.

The aim of the Directive was to promote research and development in the field of biotechnology in the European Community by securing effective and harmonized protection of biotechnological inventions. The Directive also sought to avoid creating a separate body of law by determining both the subject matter eligible for patenting and the subject matter that was to be excluded from patent protection.

The European Parliament rejected an earlier text of the Directive in March 1995 because it wanted the wording of the Directive to give a more prominent

---

[219]   Matthew Rimmer, 'The Attack of the Clones: Patent Law and Stem Cell Research', *Journal of Law and Medicine*, 10:4 (2003), 448–507.

[220]   EPC, Article 53 (a).

[221]   U.S. Patent 5843780 – Primate Embryonic Stem Cells, issued on 1 December 1998.

[222]   Erika Check, 'Canada Stops Harvard's Oncomouse in its Tracks', *Nature*, 420 (12 December 2002), 593.

[223]   Directive 98/44/EC on Biotechnological Inventions.

role to ethics and morality within patent law.[224] A compromise text was eventually adopted that included a 'morality clause' in the form of Article 6:

> Inventions shall be considered unpatentable when their commercial exploitation could be contrary to *ordre public* or morality.[225]

In fact, the final text was oriented towards the affirmation of ethical principles by excluding the patentability of inventions linked with ethically sensitive issues. As already mentioned, the human body and the simple discovery of one of its elements[226] as well as processes for cloning human beings or processes for modifying the germ line genetic identity of human beings and uses of human embryos for industrial or commercial purposes[227] were to be considered unpatentable as their exploitation went contrary to *ordre public* or public morality. Recital 38 of the Directive also notes that the list of unpatentable inventions is not exhaustive and all processes whose use went against human dignity were also to be excluded from patentability.[228]

The Directive was not well received by several EU member states. In fact the Netherlands, supported by Italy and Norway, challenged the legal validity of the Directive the same year it was adopted before the European Court of Justice.[229] One of the principal issues contested by the Netherlands was the patentability of isolated parts of the human body as provided by Article 5(2) of the Directive.[230] According to the Netherlands, the Directive reduced living human matter to a means to an end and undermined human dignity. However, the Court rejected the plea on the grounds that as only inventions which combine a natural element with a technical process enabling it to be isolated or produced for an industrial application can be the subject of a patent, it is logical to infer that it is only an element of the human body that is part of a product that is in actual fact, patentable and conversely, such an element of the human body, in its natural state, cannot be appropriated.

While the deadline for implementing the Directive into the national laws of the member states was 31 July 2000, Italy, Luxembourg, Latvia and Lithuania

---

[224]   Plomer and others, *Stem Cell Patents*, p. 20.

[225]   Directive 98/44/EC, Article 6.

[226]   Ibid., Article 5.

[227]   Directive 98/44/EC, Article 6.

[228]   Ibid., Recital 38.

[229]   Case C – 377/98 *Netherlands* v. *European Parliament and Council* [2001] ECR 1-07079.

[230]   Directive 98/44/EC, Article 5(2).

had still not implemented the Directive by the stipulated time. And while all member states have by now incorporated the Directive in their national laws, there are serious discrepancies in the way a number of member states have chosen to interpret the wording of the Directive, especially in relation to the exclusion of the uses of human embryos under Article 6 (2) c.[231]

On 16 June 1999, the Administrative Council of the European Patent Organization decided to transpose the wording of the provisions of the Directive into the EPC in the form of amendments to the EPC Implementing Regulations in order to ensure the effective implementation of the Directive. As a result, a new chapter, *Biotechnological Inventions*, comprising Rules 23 b–e,[232] was adopted as part of the Implementing Regulations. Also, with Article 164 (1) of the EPC, the Implementing Regulations became an integral part of the EPC and therefore equally binding on the EPO's Boards of Appeal[233] and on national courts. Hence, for the practical application of the EPC, only the interpretation of its provisions as laid down in its Implementing Regulations are binding and as the overwhelming majority of biotech patent applications in Europe are filed with the EPO, this means that practically all patents are issued according to the principles set forth in the Directive.

In a workshop held in June of 2001, organized by the Organization for Economic Cooperation and Development,[234] a number of concerns were identified as being responsible for the hesitancy on the part of several EU member states in adopting the Directive. Like the concerns raised with the publication of the EU Database Directive of 1996, the concerns expressed in relation to the 1998 Directive were focussed on the type of legal protection that the Directive provided to patent holders. They included the dependency that will inevitably result from DNA patents in general and from undue broad patent claims. More specifically, the main issues of concern were centred on: (i) the reluctance of researchers to enter fields with already patented genes; (ii) genetic testing and monopolistic genetic testing practices and (iii) royalty stacking and the accompanying legal disputes. It is feared that the protection provided by the Directive may, like

---

[231] Ibid., Article 6 (2).

[232] EPC, Rules 23b – 23e, 29 (6).

[233] Ibid., Article 23 (2).

[234] Joseph Strauss, 'Product Patents on Human DNA Sequences', in *Perspectives on Properties of the Human Genome Project* (Amsterdam: Elsevier Academic Press, 2003), p. 67.

the Database Directive, stifle biomedical research and as a consequence act as an obstacle towards the improvement of medical care.

The Directive draws a clear distinction between the unpatentability of the human body in its natural state and the isolation of elements from the human body that could constitute a patentable invention as long as the criteria of novelty, inventive step and industrial application are satisfied. Under Article 5 (1)[235] the Directive excludes the patentability of the human embryo and although there is no specific qualification as to whether the exclusion applies to the human embryo in the natural state or in vitro or both, it would appear that the exclusion is to be understood in the broad sense because in the final text, the qualification that no patents should be issued on the human embryo 'in its natural state' present in an earlier text was removed.[236] Hence the exclusion of Article 5 (1) extends to in vitro human embryos irrespective of the manner how they were originally created.[237] Some member states, such as the UK, for example, have gone further by interpreting Article 5 (1) as excluding also from patentability totipotent hESCs[238] in virtue of the fact that once they are isolated, they can be used for implantation and actualize their potential to develop into a human embryo. However, the exclusion does not extend to pluripotent hESCs[239] as, unlike totipotent hESCs, they lack the potential to develop into any cell found in the human embryo. Accordingly their isolation from the human body can constitute a patentable invention according to Article 5(2). As such these cells can only be excluded from patentability on the basis of the morality clause of Article 6.[240]

The problem with Article 5 is that while in paragraph (1) it is stated that the human body, at the various stages of its formation and development, and the simple discovery of one of its elements, including the sequence or partial se-

---

[235]   Directive 98/44/EC, Article 5 (10).

[236]   Opinion of the Economic and Social Committee on the 'Proposal for a European Parliament and Council Directive on the Legal Protection of Biotechnological Inventions'. OJ, C295 of 7 October 1996.

[237]   Plomer and others, *Stem Cell Patents*, pp. 66–68.

[238]   Totipotent stem cells have the potential to develop into any cell found in the human embryo.

[239]   Pluripotent stem cells have the potential to develop into almost any cell of the human embryo but not all. These pluripotent stem cells are found in the Inner Cell Mass within the blastocyst that is formed roughly four days after fertilization. Unlike totipotent stem cells, pluripotent stem cells lack the potential to develop into the placenta and other tissues that are vital for foetal development.

[240]   Directive 98/44/EC, Article 6.

quence of a gene, cannot constitute patentable inventions, paragraph (2) considers as patentable invention the isolation of any elements from the human body or otherwise produced by means of a technical process, including the sequence or partial sequence of a gene, even though the structure of the element may be identical to that of a natural element. Article 6 appears to be an extension of Article 5 in the sense that it provides a non-exhaustive list of inventions that are unpatentable because they go against *ordre public*.

Albeit the legal system of the EU is grounded in the principles of European law, the Union is authorized to function only strictly within certain parameters in virtue of the fact that it is made up of several member states with different cultures and sensibilities in relation to ethical issues.[241] For example, the EU can only exercise its authority within the spaces left to it by the treaties signed within the Union and subject to the principles of subsidiarity and proportionality that are enshrined within the constitutional texture of the Union. In other words, the EU must at all times show great respect towards the national identities of its member states. Accordingly, both the European Convention on Human Rights and the Jurisprudence of the European Court of Human Rights insist that in the implementation of the Directives adopted by the EU, great care must be taken to ensure that the national constitutional traditions and identities of the different member states are given due consideration.[242] On the level of protection and rights to be conferred on the human embryo, both the European Convention on Human Rights and the Jurisprudence of the European Court of Human Rights, while supporting the EU's original aim behind Directive 98/44/EC, namely to secure effective and harmonized protection of biotechnological inventions throughout the EU member states, are in agreement with the European Court of Justice ruling in the Netherlands case that member states are to be granted a wide margin of discretion in the interpretation of the general exclusion clause in Article 6 (1) in the light of the diversity of national cultures in Europe on morally sensitive issues. The matter is made more complex by the fact that the legal situation concerning the concept of embryo is very unclear within the EU. For example, while the embryo is protected by law from conception in Ireland, most

---

[241]   Plomer and others, *Stem Cell Patents*, pp. 36–40.
[242]   Ibid., pp. 40–49.

other countries only acknowledge the embryo a legal value from its fourteenth day of development.[243]

So, while the EPO is not bound by European Community law, still, the member states of the European Community are bound by European Community law and the contracting states to the EPC should have a national patent law in line with the EPC. At the same time, although the European Patent Office is not bound by European Community law, it is bound to act within the parameters of European Community law as there is no mechanism that can solve any disputes that may arise between the two institutions.

The main bone of contention remains the morality clause of the Directive 98/44/EC that is open to divergent interpretations, especially in relation to the different sensibilities to moral issues as reflected by the different cultures of the member states. Things are not made easier by the fact that one of the founding principles of European Community law is that the Community respects the national identities of the member states. In fact, such an approach was reflected in the Netherlands case[244] where the European Court of Justice ruled that member states are to be granted a wide margin of discretion in interpreting the morality clause of the Directive 98/44/EC. So, while Directive 98/44/EC establishes policy standards for EU member states, it does not have the force of national law![245]

At the same time, the European Court of Justice has ruled in the Italy case that unlike with Article 6 (1) which allows a wide margin of discretion in the implementation of moral exclusions, no such discretion is allowed in relation to the implementation of Article 6 (2) as the criteria employed to compile the list of inventions that go against *ordre public* were intended to reflect a moral consensus among EU member states on these sensitive moral issues. The ruling of the European Court of Justice reflects the Community Legislator's wording of Article 6 (2) which, on the one hand, excludes from patentability certain uses of the human embryo and on the other hand does not render unpatentable uses of the human embryo that are legal in some member states.

---

[243]   European Group on Ethics in Science and New Technologies to the European Commission, *Opinion on the Ethical Aspects of Patenting Inventions Involving Human Stem Cells*, Opinion Number 16, 7 May 2002.

[244]   Case C-377/98 *Netherlands* v. *European Parliament and Council* [2001] ECR 1-07079.

[245]   B. Knoppers, M. Hirtle and K. Glass, 'Commercialization of Genetic Research and Public Policy', *Science*, 286 (1999), 2277–78.

1.6 The Stem-Cell Market

The credibility of the EPO was put to the test when University of Wisconsin researcher James Thomson and his co-workers took the scientific community by surprise in November 1998 after they reported that they had isolated and cultured human embryonic stem cells. The cells were isolated from embryos that had been created at an IVF clinic and later donated to research. Thomson was the first researcher to turn hES cells into primitive blood cells using an intuitive, all natural approach that took advantage of the communicative value of the cells. Thomson cleverly co-cultured hES cells with adult blood cells to see if the adult cells would guide hES cells and in fact they did.[246]

Five-day-old hES cells were used that, as stated earlier, came from spare IVF-clinic embryos destined to be thrown away. The advantage in using these five-day-old hES cells was that they had the capability, unlike older foetal cells, to proliferate endlessly with the result that scientists were no longer preoccupied with the need to seek more cells and they could also use standardized doses. These cells were also more potent, pliable and responsive.[247]

Thomson's path-breaking work led to two important patents in the US, the first on a purified preparation of primate embryonic stem cells and the second on a method for producing these stem cell lines.[248] The patents were issued to Thomson as inventor who assigned them immediately to the Wisconsin Alumni Research Foundation (WARF) which handled intellectual property generated at Thomson's workplace, the University of Wisconsin, Madison. These patents were highly criticized for several reasons, chief among them that they involved human embryonic stem cells, that they impeded access for research and that they should never have been granted in the first place for moral reasons.

But a patent application by WARF,[249] relating to cultures of primate, including human embryonic stem cells was refused, in July 2004, by the Examining Division of the EPO on the grounds that it went against public morality. WARF appealed the decision of the Examining Division and the matter was referred to the Technical Board of Appeal on 3 September 2004 and on the 18

---

[246] Cynthia Fox, *Cell of Cells: The Global Race to Capture and Control Stem Cell* (New York: W.W. Norton & Company, 2007), p. 85.

[247] Ibid., pp. 361–62.

[248] J.A. Thomson and others, 'Embryonic Stem Cell Lines Derived from Human Blastocysts', *Science,* 282 (6 November 1998), 1145–47.

[249] European Patent Application No. 96903521.1 – Primate Embryonic Stem Cells (1995).

November 2004, WARF presented the Grounds of Appeal. The Enlarged Board of Appeal[250] of the EPO was then asked to consider the patentability of hES cells following a referral by the Technical Board of Appeal of the EPO.[251] The question facing the Enlarged Board of Appeal was whether the exploitation of hES cells was contrary to morality as Article 53 (a) of the EPC provides that European patents shall not be granted in respect of

> Inventions the publication or exploitation of which would be contrary to *ordre public* or morality, provided that the exploitation shall not be deemed to be so contrary merely because it is prohibited by law or regulation in some or all of the contracting states.[252]

The Enlarged Board of Appeal also has a guide in Rule 23d (c) of the EPC which states:

> Under Article 53 (a), European patents shall not be granted in respect of biotechnological inventions which, in particular, concern the following:
>
> a)   uses of human embryos for industrial or commercial purposes.[253]

To add to the complexity of the case, in situations where the articles and rules come into conflict,[254] it is the articles which prevail. So, Rule 23d (c) is only valid when it does not conflict with the morality clause of Article 53 (a). This rule was adopted by the European Patent Organization, as were all the other rules, when it sought to adopt the regulations on patentability accepted by the

---

[250]   Points of law can be referred to the Enlarged Board of Appeal by the President of the European Patent Office and by the Technical Boards of Appeal of the European Patent Office. No further appeal can be lodged against decisions of the Enlarged Board of Appeal.

[251]   The Enlarged Board of Appeal is responsible for ensuring the uniform application of patent law under the European Patent Convention and its decisions are binding in relation to patent practice at the European Patent Office.

[252]   Convention on the Grant of European Patents (European Patent Convention), 12th Ed. (Munich: European Patent Office, 2006).

[253]   This Rule entered into force on 1 September 1999 and corresponds to Article 6 (2) (c) of the EU Directive on the Legal Protection of Biotechnological Inventions (Directive 98/44/EC) which requires that this Article 'does not affect inventions for therapeutic or diagnostic purposes which are applied to the human embryo and are useful to it'. However, this exception does not apply in this case since obtaining stem cells from an embryo involves the destruction of the embryo and so the intervention cannot be said to be useful to it.

[254]   EPC, Article 164 (2).

EU member states in 1998 in the Directive on the Legal Protection of Biotechnological Inventions without having to revise patent law as this would have required ratification by all European member states party to the EPC.[255]

The problem with the Thomson patent application is that neither the EPC nor the Directive on the Legal Protection of Biotechnological Inventions deals specifically with human embryonic stem cells. The only references are to be found in Rule 23 d (c) of the EPC and Recital 42 of the Directive.[256] While Rule 23 d (c) provides that the use of human embryos for industrial or commercial purposes is to be excluded from patentability, Recital 42 of the Directive states that such an exclusion does not effect inventions for therapeutic or diagnostic purposes which are applied to the human embryo and are useful to it.

Rule 23 e (1)[257] of the EPC talks specifically about the human body and only indirectly about the human embryo when it is incorporated in the rule as a particular stage of the human body. The rule states categorically that the human body, at the various stages of its development and hence comprising the stage when it is a human embryo, cannot constitute a patentable invention. Recital 21,[258] however, of the Directive provides that an element isolated from the human body or otherwise produced is not to be excluded from patentability if it is the result of technical processes which humans alone are capable of putting into practice and which nature is incapable of accomplishing by itself. Finally, Rule 23 e (2)[259] of the EPC provides that isolated cells may constitute a patentable invention as long as the cells were isolated by means of a technical process even though this structure may be identical to that of the natural element. Recital 16[260] then provides that germ cells are not patentable, in line with the fundamental principles at the basis of patent law meant to safeguard the dignity and integrity of the person.

A more direct approach to the question of human embryonic stem cells was adopted by European Group of Ethics (EGE) when the Group published Opinion 16 on the *Ethical Aspects of Patenting Inventions Involving Human Stem Cells.*

---

[255] Sigrid Sterckx and Julian Cockbain, 'Patenting Human Embryonic Stem Cells', *PropEur* 3 (Winter 2006), Supplement. <http://www.propeur.bham.ac.uk/Newsletter%20Vol%203%20Supplement.pdf> [accessed on 10 June 2008]
EPC, Rule 23 d (c).

[256] Directive 98/44/EC on Biotechnological Inventions, Recital 42.

[257] EPC, Rule 23 e (1).

[258] Directive 98/44/EC, Recital 21.

[259] EPC, Rule 23 e (2).

[260] Directive 98/44/EC, Recital 16.

For the EGE, there is no specific ethical obstacle to allowing the patentability of products and processes involving human embryonic stem cells whatever their source, as long as the criteria of patentability, namely, novelty, inventive step and industrial application are maintained. So, while unmodified isolated stem cells and unmodified stem cell lines are considered unpatentable subject matter by the EGE, the contrary is true for human embryonic stem cell lines that have been modified by in vitro treatments or genetically modified in such a manner that they acquire characteristics for specific industrial application. In its Opinion, the EGE, while recognizing that the derivation of human stem cells raises different ethical concerns, depending on the source of stem cells, it held that these ethical concerns were adequately addressed by the 1998 EU Directive on the Legal Protection of Biotechnological Inventions, when the Directive stressed that processes that could lead to uses of human embryos for industrial or commercial purposes were contrary to *ordre public* and morality and so could not be patented.[261] However, included in Opinion 16 of the EGE was the *Dissident Opinion* of Professor Gunter Virt who objected to the EGE's position that there is no specific ethical obstacle to allowing the patentability of products and processes involving human embryonic stem cells, whatever their source, as long as the criteria of patentability, namely, novelty, inventive step and industrial application are maintained.

The decision of the Examining Division to reject the Thomson patent has been contested by WARF on a question of interpretation of Rule 23 d (c) in conjunction with Article 53 (a) of the EPC. For the Examining Division, the provisions of Rule 23d (c) in conjunction with Article 53 (a), although not directed exclusively to the claimed subject-matter of the patent application, are more broadly concerned with inventions that use human embryos for industrial or commercial purposes and so are considered unpatentable. The invention relies exclusively on the use of human embryos and the generated cell cultures do not serve any therapeutic or diagnostic purpose useful to the embryo and so in this case, Recital 42 does not apply. With regards to the subject-matter claimed by the patent application, while it discloses a method for the preparation of embryonic stem cells derived from primate blastocysts with specific reference to the preparation of ES cells from rhesus monkey and marmoset, it also discloses that the same technique will be used to isolate and grow human ES cells, whose source would be spare hES cells produced in IVF procedures. The original application, though primarily directed to cell cultures, rather than to a method for

---

[261]   Directive 98/44/EC, Article 6.

the generation of these cell cultures, failed to specify how these cell cultures could be produced and so it was logical for the Examining Division to extrapolate that (i) the disclosed cell cultures of embryonic stem cells, (ii) the methods for generating them and (iii) the use of an embryo as a starting material were to be taken as one unified invention. Accordingly, as the patent application appeared to enable the use of human embryos for the generation of hES cells, such a procedure fell under the provisions of Rule 23 d (c) of the EPC which excludes from patentability inventions that concern the use of human embryos for industrial or commercial purposes.[262]

The position of the Examining Division reflected the *Dissenting Opinion* of Professor Gunter Virt from the EGE.[263] Virt expressed his dissent at allowing the patenting of processes and products that use material resulting from destroyed human embryos. He expressed his concern that the patenting of human embryonic stem cells and human embryonic stem cell lines contradicted the dignity of the human embryo as a human being with the derived right to life since the attainment of these products and processes used the human embryo as source material. He also expressed his concern that the patenting of human embryonic stem cells and human embryonic stem cell lines would push research towards embryonic stem cells with the result that research using non-embryonic stem cells such as adult stem cells is sidelined.[264]

When the WARF patent was initially lodged with the EPO, the Examining Division had also explored the possibility that a reading of Directive 98/44/EC Recital 42[265] could have a bearing on the case. This recital provides that the exclusion from patentability does not effect inventions for therapeutic or diagnostic purposes which are applied to the human embryo and are useful to it. However, the conclusions of the Examining Division were such that the generation of hES cell cultures could not in any way be considered as serving therapeutic

---

[262] The decision of the Examining Division to refuse the application was based on the grounds that the subject matter of claims 1-7, 9 and 10 is not patentable under Article 53 (a) and Rule 23 d (c) EPC.

[263] European Group on Ethics in Science and New Technologies to the European Commission, *Opinion on the Ethical Aspects of Patenting Inventions Involving Human Stem Cells*, Opinion Number 16, 7 May 2002.

[264] Prof. Gunter Virt, 'Dissident Opinion', in *Opinion on the Ethical Aspects of Patenting Inventions Involving Human Stem Cells*, by European Group on Ethics in Science and New Technologies to the European Commission, Opinion Number 16, 7 May 2002.

[265] The Directive 98/44/EC can be used as a supplementary means of interpretation of the provisions of the EPC concerning the patenting of biotechnological inventions.

or diagnostic purposes useful to the human embryo when, after having been used as the source of hES cells, these human embryos simply ceased to exist!

The objections raised by WARF on the conclusions reached by the Examining Division centred on two main points, namely that the interpretation of Rule 23 d (c)[266] was incorrect as the claimed subject matter related only to cell cultures and not to any method of production of these cell cultures and that if the interpretation adopted by the Examining Division was taken to be correct then this would mean that all downstream products such as growth factors or other important medicinal products, isolated from human embryonic tissues or in any way traceable back to human embryonic tissues, would also be excluded from patentability with devastating consequences for future biotechnological inventions.

The Enlarged Board of Appeal, to which the case was referred by the Technical Board of Appeal in 2005, after the decision of the Examining Division was appealed by WARF, gave a final ruling on 25 November 2008.[267] This ruling reiterated the decision of the Examining Division of 13 July 2004 that rejected the WARF/Thomson patent application on the grounds that it fell within the exception to patentability of Article 53 (a) and Rule 28 (c) of the EPC.[268] However, although the Enlarged Board of Appeal banned the patentability of inventions that could only be exploited through the destruction of human embryos, it did not go into the issue of the possible patentability of human stem cell cultures. In fact, while many have interpreted the Enlarged Board of Appeal's ruling as including a ban on the patentability of human embryonic stem cells, others have argued that this is not the case and that in the future, it would be possible for the EPO to grant patents on human stem cells if they are not obtained by the destruction of human embryos because in this way, the exclusion clause of Rule 28 (c) will be surpassed in its entirety!

The general question of human stem cell patentability had already been raised with the European patent granted to the University of Edinburgh in 1999 for a method of isolating and/or enriching and/or selectively propagating desired animal stem cells.[269] When the application was filed, 14 parties opposed the

---

[266]   EPC, Rule 23 d (c).

[267]   Decision of the Enlarged Board of Appeal of 25 November 2008.

[268]   The Enlarged Board of Appeal based its ruling on the relevant provisions of the European Patent Convention (Article 53 (a) and Rule 28 (c)) and on the EU Biotechnology Directive (98/44/EC) that was implemented in the European Patent Convention in 1999.

[269]   European Patent No. 0 695 351.

granting of the patent, citing among other reasons that the claimed subject matter was contrary to the morality provisions of Article 53 (a) of the EPC.[270] The Opposition Division of the EPO was faced with the question of whether the provisions of Rule 23 d (c) concerning the uses of human embryos for industrial or commercial purposes were to be interpreted in a broad or narrow fashion. The conclusion of the Opposition Division was that only a broad interpretation of the Rule was appropriate given the provisions of the Directive on the Legal Protection of Biotechnological Inventions[271] and so an amended patent[272] was granted for a method of isolating and/or enriching and/or selectively propagating desired animal stem cells other than human embryonic stem cells. The position of the Opposition Division, based on the aims of the Directive 98/44/EC, was that not only was the use of human embryos to be excluded from patentability but also the use of human embryonic stem cells retrieved by the destruction of human embryos. On the other hand, amended claims were allowed by the Opposition Division on any pluripotent or multipotent stem cells which could be isolated from adults or umbilical cord blood or from foetal tissues obtained after pregnancy termination.[273]

1.7 Patents and the Pursuit of Scientific Progress

The metaphor, *tragedy of the commons* was first used by Garrett Hardin in 1968 in order to explain how people are responsible for such problems as overpopulation, air pollution and species extinction by overusing resources that are held in common without any incentive to conserve.[274] However, the recent proliferation of intellectual property rights in biomedical research is producing another form of tragedy, this time the '*tragedy of the anti-commons*' as people underuse scarce resources because too many patent owners block each other. Several phenomena contribute to the rise of an anti-commons in biotechnology but the main causes are related to the licensing of materials and methods that could prevent researchers from making new discoveries or developing new products.[275]

---

[270] Helen Bearley, The Patentability of Stem Cells, 2008. <http://www.elkfife.com/view_article.php?id=70> [accessed on 2 January 2009]

[271] Directive 98/44/EC.

[272] European Patent No. B1 – 695351.

[273] Bearley, 'The Patentability of Stem Cells'.

[274] Garrett Hardin, 'The Tragedy of the Commons', *Science*, 162 (1968), 1243–48.

[275] Resnik, 'A Biotechnology Patent Pool'.

The *tragedy of the anti-commons* was started some twenty years ago when in the US, research institutions such as the National Institutes of Health (NIH) and major universities created technology transfer offices to patent and license their discoveries. This marked a shift in policy from the traditional knowledge of academia, generally governed by norms facilitating full and rapid publication, disclosure, and sharing of knowledge with a minimum of restrictions on other scientists after research material is shared.[276] In return, scientists were rewarded for publishing their research and awarded recognition for scientific priority. In contrast, with the private sector, research knowledge has always been protected by exclusive intellectual property rights that gave scientists the right to prevent other scientists from using their patented material. With the *Bayle-Dole Act* of 1980 which streamlined the rules for academic patenting, many research institutions began to publish and patent ideas simultaneously. At the same time commercial biotechnology firms have emerged finding a new lucrative niche in the biotechnology industry by straddling the traditional academia of research institutions such as universities on the one hand and the product market of pharmaceutical companies on the other. In recent years, upstream research in the biomedical science is most likely to be private, supported by private funds, carried out in a private institution or privately appropriated through patents, trade secrecy or agreements that restrict the use of materials or data. As a result we have seen a spiral of overlapping patent claims in the hands of different owners with researchers having to negotiate dozens or even hundreds of licenses that they might require to develop a new product. This inevitably creates a *tragedy of the anti-commons* situation where each upstream patent allows its owner to set up another tollbooth on the road to product development, adding to the cost and slowing the pace of downstream biomedical innovation.[277] For example, when James Thomson succeeded in isolating and culturing human embryonic stem cells, the University of Wisconsin not only had material rights to the cell lines its researchers generated but, as a result of patent applications filed by Thomson on his discoveries, owned property rights that encompassed both Thomson's stem cells and the core techniques to develop them. As a result, the University of Wisconsin has controlled the stem cell market by imposing up-front license fees for the use of any patented material or technology. Furthermore, it charged

---

[276]   Fiona Murray, 'The Stem-Cell Market—Patents and the Pursuit of Scientific Progress', *The New England Journal of Medicine*, 356 (2007), 2341–43.

[277]   Heller and Eisenberg, 'Can Patents Deter Innovation?', pp. 698–701.

royalties for the sale of any products derived from the licensed technology and the transfer of any material for research purposes or publication by third parties.[278] It was only in January 2007 that the University of Wisconsin eased restrictions on stem-cell transfers among researchers and began permitting, without the need to pay a license fee, industry-sponsored research on stem cells in academic institutions.[279]

1.8 Who Owns You?

One-fifth of human genes have already been claimed as US Intellectual Property. But should anyone own our genes? And what happens when gene ownership can drastically prevent the advancement of life-saving cures?

The US Patent Office's most controversial patents are on BRCA1 and BRCA2, both linked to the high risks of ovarian and breast cancer. They are now owned by Myriad Genetics Laboratories. In 1996, Myriad Genetics developed and began marketing a predictive test for the presence of possible cancerous-mutations: the 'BRCAnalysis' test. The price of the test was US$3,000 but the company promised that it would eventually drop the price to US$300. This never happened because its patent holder had the right to stop any other party from duplicating the patented sequences. This single test accounted for over 80% of Myriad Genetics' multibillion dollar business.

In 2009, the American Civil Liberties Union (ACLU), Tania Simoncelli, who is the organization science officer, decided to challenge the patenting of human genes on legal grounds. She went to the ACLU where Chris Hansen, had been an institutional knowledge and had insights. Together, there were the representative of 20 medical organisations, geneticists, women's health groups, and patients unable to be screened due to the prohibitive patents. The ACLU's position was that Myriad's patents violated the patent law on the issue of patent-eligibility.

The case went before the Supreme Court. By 3 June 2013 it was declared that the Myriad patents were invalid because they did not create or alter any of the genetic information encoded in the BRCA1 and BRCA2 genes. The location and order of the nucleotides existed in nature before Myriad found them. The company simply discovered what was already there and did not create anything new.

---

[278]   Murray, 'The Stem-Cell Market', p. 2342.

[279]   Ibid.

There is no worldwide consensus on whether parts of the human genome should be granted Intellectual Property protection. The Myriad patents should alert us to the injustice of having a pharmaceutical company make money out of cancer predictive tests that could cost 10 times less than what is charged. The same patents stifled diagnostic testing and research that could have led to cures as well as limiting women's options regarding their medical care in Malta as in all other parts of the world. There are various international and regional agreements that have described the human genome as being part of humanity's 'common heritage', including the 1998 UN Declaration on the Human Genome and Human Rights. The Myriad patents controversy has shown that gene patenting does not work to stimulate more research—one of the prime arguments Big Pharma uses. It is time to explore other avenues that will both promote scientific progress and technological development but at the same time protect the special nature of human genes that make us who we are. No one should own our genes— they should be exploited in the interest of everyone.

Professional organizations however are opposed to gene patents because they threaten biomedical research and patient care. This is the view of both the American College of Medical Genetics and the College of American Pathologists, to cite two examples. The World Medical Association has gone even a step further by considering human genes to be part of mankind's common heritage and has urged medical organizations around the world to lobby against gene patenting.[280] The consideration here is that it is immoral to patent DNA because the human genome is our common heritage and therefore should not be privately owned or commercialized. Based on the Roman Law tradition of *jus utendi et abutendi*,[281] the patent system gives an exclusive property right to the inventor to 'use and misuse' the work already started on his invention. The patent holder can choose to exclude others from making, using or commercializing his or her invention.[282] For this reason, the patent system is incompatible with the principle of common heritage of mankind.[283] Using Grotian terms based on Roman Law, the human genome, as *res communis*, cannot be owned by anyone, must be available for use by everyone and can never be appropriated by anyone. The patenting system considers the human genome as public property or *res*

---

[280]   Andrews, 'Genes and Patent Policy', pp. 803–08.

[281]   Elizabeth Mann Borgese (ed.), *Pacem in Maribus* (New York: Dodd, Mead & Company, 1972), pp. 161–65.

[282]   Patent and Trademark Office, *General Information Concerning Patents* (Washington D.C.: Patent and Trademark Office, 1999).

[283]   Resnik, *Owning the Genome*, p. 77.

publica which can become *res extra commercium* when what does not form part of the estate of an individual can be appropriated and become part of an individual estate. Considering that the human genome consists of genes and genetic information on the life of humanity, it stands to reason that the human genome should be considered a common resource. Considering that the human genome constitutes the distinctive element specific to each individual as a component of his or her uniqueness, it stands to reason that it cannot be appropriated.[284] In an *amicus* brief[285] of the Peoples Business Commission, the Commission, while arguing that the US Congress never intended to allow the patenting of living organisms, stated that:

> We have paid some high prices for the technological conquest of nature, but none perhaps so high as the intellectual and spiritual costs of seeing nature as mere material for our manipulation, exploitation and transformation.[286]

Inspired by the morality clause of the EPC, Timothy Caulfied and Richard Gold have proposed to use the patent system itself as a moral tollbooth[287] for evaluating whether patents comply with ethical and social standards. As most companies and many inventors use the patent system before they commercialize their invention, the patent application can be used to trigger an ethical review which would have the authority to withhold patents for breach of ethical standards by specifying certain types of activity rather than certain types of invention that can defy these standards. So, an activity could theoretically render the commercial sale of an invention ethically unacceptable, as happened with the Thomson patents in Europe.

---

[284] Reimer, Tanya, *New Property and Global Governance: The Common Heritage of Mankind* (submitted by Tanya Reimer on 24 April 2007 to Dr. O'Brien in partial completion of Global Governance) <http://www.tanya.peatt.net/published/property_global_gov_chh.pdf> [accessed on 10 July 2008]

[285] These amicus briefs are documents that are filed in court by individuals and groups who are not directly linked to the case in court but feel that with the information they have in their possession they can assist the court in deciding on the matter at hand.

[286] Peoples Business Commission, *Appellate Brief of Peoples' Business Commission as Amici Curiea in Support of the Petitioner in 'Diamond* v *Chakrabarty'*, WL 2005 (13 December 1979).

[287] E. Richard Gold and Timothy Caulfield, 'The Moral Tollbooth: A Method that makes use of the Patent System to Address Ethical Concerns in Biotechnology', *Lancet*, 359 (2002), 2268–70.

The EGE was thinking on the same lines when in its Opinion on the *Ethical Aspects of Patenting Involving Human Stem Cells*, it proposed that the recommendation of Article 7 of the 1998 EU Directive which delegates to the EGE the task to 'evaluate all ethical aspects of biotechnology' could be understood as requiring not only a general evaluation of biotechnology, as the Article would imply, but also specific ethical evaluations in the course of the examination of patent applications.[288] These ethical evaluations could become part of the review process of the EPO, carried out by advisory panels of independent experts set up for the purpose.[289]

This study has the goal of returning the human genome to being *res communis* from *res extra commercium* and the proposition to make patents a moral tollbooth could be the first step towards achieving this end. In the next chapter of our study, we propose to use the lessons learned from Arvid Pardo to make 'non-appropriation'[290] the basis for benefit-sharing of the human genome in the interests of all humankind. This will involve a radical overhaul of the patent system since the exclusive proprietary rights which it gives patentees are incompatible with the concept of common heritage which requires that all scientific research in the area of genetics be freely and openly disseminated to all those who express a genuine interest in it. We will be proposing a model of governance of the human genome in the form of an International Human Genome Authority (IHGA) on the same lines as the International Seabed Authority established by the Law of the Sea Convention of 1982. The review process of the EPO discussed above would be one operational arm, of the IHGA, for the member states of the EU. Other existing organizational structures such as the United States Patent and Trademark Office (USPTO) can also be retained but the *modus operandi* of these organizations will be changed in such a manner that *community interests* take precedence over *individual interests.*

---

[288]   Directive 98/44/EC, Article 7.

[289]   European Group on Ethics in Science and New Technologies to the European Commission, *Opinion on the Ethical Aspects of Patenting Inventions Involving Human Stem Cells*, Opinion Number 16, 7 May 2002.

[290]   Pardo, *The Common Heritage of Mankind*, pp. 41–42.

Chapter Two
Human Genome as Common Heritage

2.1 Philosophical Concept or Political Slogan?

The concept of common heritage of mankind has been the subject of intense debate in international circles since November 1967, when Arvid Pardo first proposed that the bounties of the deep seabed should be protected and regulated by a new kind of regime that was as much innovative in character as it was revolutionary in its legal implications.[291] Pardo's proposal was different from the traditional schemes of sovereignty and freedom that applied to territorial sea and the high seas, respectively. The common heritage of mankind was to be a new form of common ownership, in a word, an alternative to the classical Roman Law concept of *res communis*, rather than a contemporary version or extension of it.[292] In fact, at a *Pacem in Maribus* Seminar in Rhode Island in 1970, Pardo had said:

> ...we did not think it advisable to use the 'property'—not because I had anything against property—and I don't express any opinion as to the desirability or nondesirability of this ancient institution—but I thought it was not wise to use the word property...Property is a form of power. Property as we have it from ancient Romans implies the *jus utendi et abutendi* (right to use and misuse). Property implies and gives excessive emphasis to just one aspect: resource exploitation and benefit therefrom.[293]

The same concerns Pardo had about the use of the term 'property' as applied to the deep seabed and the ocean floor are equally applicable to the human genome. To Pardo, 'property' implied power with the Roman implication of *jus utendi et abutendi*—it is the same Roman Law tradition that is at the basis of the patent system which gives the patentee an exclusive property right to pursue or not pursue work already started on his or her invention.[294] It is principally for this

---

[291] Tullio Scovazzi, The Concept of Common Heritage of Mankind and the Resources of the Seabed Beyond the Limits of National Jurisdiction. <http://www.iadb.org/.../Seminario_AUS-PINTAL_2006_04_Scovazzi.pdf> [accessed on 20 April 2007]

[292] Kemal Baslar, *The Concept of the Common Heritage of Mankind in International Law* (The Hague: Martinus Nijhoff Publishers, 1998), pp. 38–39.

[293] Pardo, *The Common Heritage of Mankind*, pp. x–xi.

[294] Ibid.

reason that the patent system based on the *jus utendi et abutendi* notion of property is incompatible with the concept of common heritage of mankind. The human genome, as common heritage of mankind, must be seen as a *res communis* that cannot be owned by anyone, that must be available for use by everyone and must never become the subject of appropriation by anyone.

This *res communis* notion of property was originally applied by Hugo Grotius to the high seas after the seizure of a large Portuguese galleon in the Strait of Malacca in retaliation for Portuguese resistance to Dutch trade in the East Indies. Unfortunately, this led to the *laissez faire, laissez passer* attitude of Grotius' *Mare Liberum*[295] that continued to rule the waves for over three hundred centuries and later provided the right political platform for US President Truman to claim, in 1945, that the natural resources of the seabed and continental shelf beneath the high seas belonged to the US.[296]

The same 'hands off' approach but this time in the field of biotechnology, has given the US and other industrialized nations the opportunity to exploit the lack of proper regulation in the patenting of the human genome by putting individual rights before community rights and in so doing impeding important biomedical research. The prohibitive costs in using already patented DNA molecules is one of the major factors that are impeding research that relies on having access to these patented molecules and other products in order to develop pharmaceutical products, medical therapies and diagnostic tests.[297]

When Arvid Pardo put the concept of common heritage of mankind on the agenda of the UN General Assembly, he knew that it would not be easy to convince the industrialized member states of the political implications of the new regime of resource management that he was proposing. Chief among these political implications would be the establishment of an international authority that would manage the peaceful use and orderly exploitation of the deep seabed resources in the interests of mankind with special regard being given to the needs

---

[295] Grotius, *Freedom of the Seas*, p. 6. <http://www.oll.libertyfund.org/EBOOKS/Groti us_0049.pdf> [accessed on 22 August 2006]

[296] The continental shelf is defined as the 'seabed and subsoil of the submarine areas that extend beyond a coastal state's territorial sea throughout the natural prolongation of its land territory to the outer edge of the continental margin, or to a distance of 200 nautical miles from the baselines from which the breadth of the territorial sea is measured where the outer edge of the continental margin does not extend up to that distance'

[297] Rifkin, *The Biotech Century*, pp. 37–66.

of poor countries. The same international authority would be expected to guarantee freedom of research with the results being made freely available to all those who showed interest in the research. But in very concrete terms, this international authority would be mandated, by the international community, to assume jurisdiction as a trustee for all countries over the oceans and ocean floor with wide powers to regulate, supervise and control all activities on or under the ocean and ocean floor.[298] It was this aspect of the common heritage of mankind that was very especially important to Arvid Pardo, namely the international management of the deep seabed resources in the interests of all mankind. As we shall see, although the origin of the common heritage of mankind can be traced back to natural law and the ethic of stewardship, the international governance of the common heritage by and for all mankind was a new element which Pardo introduced and in so doing, challenged the traditional schemes of sovereignty and freedom.

Likewise, the application of the concept of common heritage of mankind to the human genome, as proposed in our study, will introduce a new model of international governance of the human genome by and for all mankind with the results of research on the human genome being registered in an international genetic databank. In this way, the individual interests of researchers will be reconciled with the community interests of all mankind. But more importantly, all uses of the genomic information registered with the new international genetic databank will be made freely available to all researchers who show interest in the information stored, subject to a reasonable fee.

As Arvid Pardo had wisely predicted, many member states of the UN did not share his concerns about the future of the seabed. The more industrialized member states were also reluctant to give up the opportunity given to them by Grotius' *laissez faire* attitude in the high seas, to appropriate for themselves the resources of the deep seabed and ocean floor. As a matter of fact, by the time Pardo's idea of common heritage of mankind was made the subject of international law with the United Nations Law of the Sea Convention (UNCLOS) of 1982,[299] much of what Arvid Pardo had wanted to achieve with the concept of

---

[298] Address by Arvid Pardo to the 22nd Session of the General Assembly of the United Nations (1967), Official Records of the General Assembly, Twenty-Second Session, Agenda Item 92, Document A/6695.

[299] Agreement Relating to the Implementation of Part XI of the United Nations Convention on the Law of the Sea of 10 December 1982, adopted by the General Assembly of the United Nations at its 48th Session on 28 July 1994. UNGA Res. 48/263.

common heritage of mankind, as he understood it, was left out of the final draft. The original formulation of the concept, as envisaged by Pardo, is to be found in the *Draft Ocean Space Treaty* that was submitted by Malta as a working paper for discussion purposes.[300] For example, whereas in the original Maltese proposal, all the natural resources, living or non-living, existing beyond the 200-mile limit were to be managed by an international institution so as to ensure the equitable sharing by all states of the benefits derived from the exploitation of these resources, UNCLOS restricted the application of the concept of common heritage of mankind solely to mineral resources.[301] Again, whereas in the Maltese draft, within the 200-mile limit, coastal states were obliged to make contributions to the international community in exchange for the financial benefits derived from the extension of their rights on the resources contained within the given area under their control, UNCLOS required coastal states to make a contribution only in relation to the exploitation of non-living resources of the continental shelf, beyond the 200-mile limit.[302]

Even still, many developed countries refused to sign the convention, citing as their main reason for not endorsing it the kind of governance that was envisaged under the common heritage of mankind regime that would, according to them, discourage mining activities by individual states and the private sector. The 1994 Implementing Agreement[303] was formulated with the precise intention to encourage these dissenting countries to come aboard and accept the UNCLOS. This was exactly what happened, with UNCLOS achieving almost universal acceptance except for the US which ironically remains the main potential deep seabed miner.[304] But universal acceptance was only attained at the cost of retaining the *laissez faire* attitude that had prevailed prior to Pardo's 1967 proposal to the General Assembly of the UN, mainly based on liberalist and market-oriented policies.

The same liberalist and market-oriented policies remain the most serious obstacle to the implementation of the Pardosian concept to the human genome.

---

[300]   Pardo, *The Common Heritage of Mankind*, pp. 381–480.
[301]   United Nations Convention of the Law of the Sea (UNCLOS), Montego Bay, 10 December 1982, Article 133.
[302]   Ibid., Article 82.
[303]   Agreement on the Implementation of Part XI of the Law of the Sea Convention, 28 July 1994.
[304]   As of 1 January 2008, the United States has not ratified the UNCLOS due to Part XI but although it is not a party to the treaty it considers many of the other provisions as binding customary law.

For example, just one week after US President Bill Clinton and UK Prime Minister Tony Blair spoke of the human genome as the 'human genetic blueprint' and acknowledged the importance of making the fundamental raw data on the human genome 'freely available to scientists everywhere',[305] the United States Patent and Trademark Office (USPTO) issued a statement saying that the US government's patent policy had remained unaffected by the Joint Statement of the two leaders.[306]

With the press release of the USPTO one week after the much publicized Joint Statement, it became clear that the two leaders had no intention of setting into motion a general overhaul of the patent system that would no longer condone the commercialization of the human genome. Their Statement turned out to be an empty political slogan that was never meant to bring about any real change in the way the human genome was being exploited by an archaic patent system that paralysed biomedical research and delayed providing people with better medical care.

So, as fate would have it, fifty years after Arvid Pardo reluctantly appointed himself, in the eyes of many, as a 'prophet of doom',[307] we find ourselves assuming the same role in the face of the reluctance of many political leaders to make the human genome a common heritage of mankind. Investing ourselves with this prophetic role on behalf of the human genome carries with it two main tasks, namely (i) to make the public understand the rich philosophical sources that have given meaning to the concept and, (ii) to set in motion the necessary political and economic machinery to change the patent system from one that serves the special interests of patentees to one that serves the interests of all mankind.

While addressing the Legal Subcommittee of the Committee on the Peaceful Uses of the Seabed and the Ocean Floor, on 10 March 1969, Pardo declared:

> Many, I know, consider me a prophet of doom and gloom because I have predicted that the present uncertain legal status of the seabed may lead to a comprehensive scramble by a few countries to appropriate for national purposes the land under the world's seas and oceans....[308]

---

[305] Bill Clinton and Tony Blair, Joint Statement by President William Clinton and Prime Minister Tony Blair of the United Kingdom (14 March 2000). <http://wwwipmall.info/hosted_resources/ippresdocs/ippd_44.htm, 14 March> [accessed on 20 March 2006]

[306] F. Gaglioti, *Wall Street and the Commercial Exploitation of the Human Genome*, quoted in Rimmer, *Intellectual Property and Biotechnology*, p. 141.

[307] Pardo, *The Common Heritage of Mankind*, p. 70.

[308] Pardo, *The Common Heritage of Mankind*, p. 70.

Pardo was aware that with the development of sophisticated technology, the developed states had acquired the means to exploit the common spaces and by employing the Roman concept of *res communis*, they were free to share the spoils of their exploits among themselves. As a result, the gap between the rich countries of the North and the poor ones of the South was bound to continue to widen in favour of the more technologically advanced countries of the North. Another factor that was of concern to Pardo was the premise of abundance on which the Roman principles of acquisition were based. After the Second World War, the enlarging world community and the increasing world population made many resources scarce and as a result the traditional concepts of ownership and entitlement theories of justice had to be re-examined.[309]

So Pardo's disappointment at the conclusion of the 1982 UNCLOS III event was no big surprise considering that the concept of common heritage of mankind became economic water shed for promoting the free exploitation of common spaces under the guise of acting in the interests of all mankind. Addressing the Legal Committee on the Peaceful Uses of the Seabed and the Ocean Floor in 1969, Pardo reminded the Committee that when the Maltese government submitted the proposal to declare the bounties of the deep sea as the common heritage of mankind, he had made it abundantly clear that urgent action was needed because:

> Need we recall that every month that passes brings the news of new encroachments in a domain that should remain intangible? If we do not proceed with speed and determination, both the area and particularly the resources that are to be explored and exploited for the benefit of all countries will be reduced almost to the vanishing point.[310]

Pardo's call for urgency underscores the fact the common heritage of mankind is first and foremost a philosophical concept meant to encourage speculation about major changes in the world such as the advent of technology and the scarcity of resources. It also has binding legal implications in so far as its provisions need to be applied by the world community in the interests of all mankind. Because of the legal implications of the concept of common heritage of mankind, Pardo has been recognized by some as a legal catalyst for making the concept of common heritage of mankind a legal principle of international law.[311] When addressing the First Committee of the General Assembly on 29 October 1968,

---

[309]   Baslar, *The Concept of the Common Heritage of Mankind in International Law*, pp. 45–46.
[310]   Pardo, *The Common Heritage of Mankind*, p. 90.
[311]   Barkenbus, *Deep Seabed Resources*, p. 32.

Pardo made it clear that the concept of common heritage of mankind was not simply an alternative to the *res communis* regime but rather a new legal principle that, if intelligently construed, could save mankind from a whole plethora of problems in the future ranging from the natural environment to our own humanness:

> For my delegation the common heritage concept is not a slogan, it is not one of a number of more or less desirable principles, but it is the very foundation of our work, the key that will unlock the door of the future.[312]

For Pardo, the concept of common heritage of mankind was not a slogan but rather a philosophical concept that had the potential to become a new legal principle of international law. But the problem that Pardo had to face and in fact we are still facing today when proposing to make the human genome the common heritage of mankind is that Treaties and General Assembly Resolutions to date have not explicitly defined the concept of common heritage of mankind. International lawyers have still to understand the real meaning of the concept in international law.[313] As Christopher Joynor remarked in his often quoted article on the legal implications of the concept of common heritage of mankind, there exists substantial confusion over the nature of the concept and its appropriate place in international law.[314] In his article, Joynor lists five different terms that are used to refer to the common heritage of mankind, namely 'concept', 'notion', 'doctrine' and 'regime', and 'ideal'.[315] The reason for this confusion is that most commentators on the common heritage of mankind seem to overlook that fact that for Arvid Pardo, the concept was essentially a philosophical concept, as explained earlier, that had legal implications and was intended to introduce a revolutionary new model of resource management. So the proper place to start work on understanding the meaning of the Pardosian term is in its roots in natural law and the stewardship ethic from which the concept of common heritage of mankind originated.

It has become imperative that the world community take recognizance of Pardo's concept of common heritage of mankind so as to be able to live up to the complex challenges that are threatening the very essence of our humanness.

---

[312] Pardo, *The Common Heritage of Mankind*, p. 64.

[313] Baslar, *The Concept of the Common Heritage of Mankind in International Law*, pp. 3–4.

[314] Joynor, 'Legal Implications of the Concept of the Common Heritage of Mankind', pp. 190–99 (p. 190).

[315] Baslar, *The Concept of the Common Heritage of Mankind in International Law*, p. 2.

The human genome is today subject to the same threat of unilateral exploitation as was the deep seabed in 1967. However, biotechnology presents a more serious threat to the human genome than technology did to the deep seabed resources because of the very nature of the human genome. The problem is that the human genome is not a thing or *res* that can be declared a *res communis* as happened with the high seas, outer space and celestial bodies. The human genome has an ontological significance that is not to be found in these three common resources. For this reason, the objectification of the human genome by biotechnology has far more serious implications than the potential exploitation of the high seas, for example. At the same time, the race to grab the bounties of the human genome appears to be no different than the race to grab the bounties of the deep seabed that Pardo feared so much in the 1960s and 70s. This is because there are many who argue that the human genome is no different from the resources of the deep seabed and therefore can be appropriated by those who have the potential to exploit it.

The question of whether the human genome should be made subject to appropriation through patenting or whether it should remain free from appropriation as a common heritage of mankind is reduced to the question of whether the human genome is the embodiment of our humanness, determining both our individuality and our species identity or whether the human genome is merely a 'blob of cells' or 'conglomeration of molecules'[316] and so reducible to a thing or *res* that can be patented? As a common heritage resource, can we equate the human genome to the deep seabed, outer space or the moon? Probably not, because the nature of the human genome is very different from the other common space areas, a fact that was underlined by Article 1 of the Universal Declaration on the Human Genome and Human Rights that proclaimed the human genome as being, 'in a symbolic sense, the heritage of humanity'.[317] Still, in proposing to make the deep seabed the common heritage of mankind, Arvid Pardo went beyond the *res communis* concept because in his eyes, the emphasis had to be on the notions of 'non-appropriation' and 'international management' rather than on the fact of 'common possession'.[318] And this is where international lawyers get stuck when it comes to finding a common definition of the common

---

[316]   David Holbrook, Medical Ethics and the Potentialities of the Living Being, *British Medical Journal (Clinical Research Edition)*, 291 (1985), 459–62 (p. 459).

[317]   Universal Declaration on the Human Genome and Human Rights, adopted by the General Conference of UNESCO at its 29th Session on 11 November 1997, Article 1.

[318]   Pardo, *The Common Heritage of Mankind*, pp. 41–42.

heritage of mankind because the radical meaning of the concept is to be found not in an alternative formulation of the *res communis* notion but in a new theory of international management by and for mankind based on the absence of property rights or non-appropriation.

As stated earlier, the concept of common heritage of mankind is not an extension of the *res* regime but a totally new concept of governance founded on natural law, inspired by the ethic of stewardship and complemented by Pardo's notion of international management. This is the philosophical understanding of the concept of common heritage of mankind that unfortunately has been absent in both national and international debates on the concept. It is the philosophical hubris in which the concept of common heritage of mankind has been nurtured and which will continue to guide our effort to make the human genome a common heritage of mankind. Albeit the human genome was declared the common heritage of mankind in 1997, unfortunately, as stated above, there remains confusion as to what is the nature of the concept and its standing in international law. These difficulties were enhanced rather than reduced by the drafters' choice of words in referring to the human genome as being, 'in a symbolic sense, the heritage of humanity'.

The human genome fundamentally is both matter and form in the sense that it is both genes and genetic information, together constituting *in-forma-tion* on the life of humanity.[319] This genomic metaphysics sees the genome as Aristotle's *eidos* which is the organizing principle inherent in every living thing.[320]

Accordingly, the relation between the human genome and the concept of common heritage of mankind must be studied from a philosophical perspective for three principal reasons, namely (i) to understand the true nature of the human genome, (ii) to clarify the Pardosian meaning of the concept of common heritage of mankind and (iii) to incorporate the concept as a legal principle in international law.

---

[319] Leon R. Kass, *Toward a More Natural Science: Biology and Human Affairs* (New York: The Free Press, 1985), pp. 253–58.

[320] Alex Mauron, 'Is the Genome the Secular Equivalent of the Soul?', *Science*, 291 (2001), 831–32.

2.2   Beneath the Surface
of the Common Heritage of Mankind

The emergence of the concept of common heritage of mankind has been one of the most extraordinary developments in recent intellectual history referred to, by different academics, as a 'political moral innovation', as a 'transcendental notion', as a 'philosophical concept' and as a 'world-changing phrase'.[321] The common heritage of mankind marked the end of positivist Westphalian international law which vested sovereignty exclusively in the monarch whose authority was founded on mandate and history. The Treaty of Westphalia[322] signed in 1648 gave rise to a number of foundational principles of international law which remained practically unchanged until Hugo Grotius, in 1609, challenged the status quo of international law with his *Mare Liberum*[323] and Arvid Pardo, in 1967, launched the concept of common heritage of mankind to protect and regulate the resources of the deep seabed and ocean floor. Both Grotius and Pardo challenged the very foundations of international law which included: (i) the sovereign state's right to use exclusive force; (ii) the right of non-intervention in internal affairs; (iii) consent as the basis of obligation for complying with international laws and (iv) diplomatic immunity.[324]

Practically all available land on Earth has been claimed by a sovereign state since the signing of the Treaty of Westphalia except for the deep seabed, the Arctic and Antarctica. And today, thirty years after the first gene patents were claimed around 1978, more than one-fifth of the almost 24,000 human genes are under patent. This deluge of genetic patents was the result of the launch of the HGP and the introduction of rapid sequencing technologies. It won't be long before most, if not all human genes, will be under patent. Pardo's concern was that the land under the world's seas and oceans does not end up appropriated by a few nations for national purposes.[325] Our concern is that patented genes are

---

[321]   Baslar, *The Concept of the Common Heritage of Mankind in International Law*, p. 7.

[322]   W. Michael Reisman, 'The Problem of Sovereignty and Human Rights in Contemporary International Law', *American Journal of International Law*, 84 (1990), 866–76.

[323]   Schakelford, Scott J., 'The Tragedy of the Common Heritage of Mankind', *Stanford Environmental Law Journal* (Stanford Public Law Working Paper No. 1407332), 27 (2008), 1–72 (p. 2).

[324]   Ibid., p. 5.

[325]   Pardo, *The Common Heritage of Mankind*, p. 70.

blocking future research, preventing medical testing and impeding further discoveries into these genes. Take for example the patents awarded to Myriad Genetics which have already been discussed earlier in this study. Public officials in the European Union, North America and Australasia decried the granting of these patents when they are blocking patient access to treatment, breast cancer research and the administration of healthcare.[326] In the absence of a comprehensive system of regulation of the human genome that does not create such an anti-commons effect that, among other things, makes researchers spend large amounts of money on complex licensing operations in order to gain access to multi-patented genes, it may be wise for the international community to consider a moratorium on any further patenting of the human genome.

Hugo Grotius was trying to fill another void in the proper regulation of common resources when he wrote his *Mare Liberum* with the purpose of establishing some form of regulation of the high seas after the taking of the Portuguese galleon by the Dutch East India Company in protest at the Spanish-Portuguese attempt to control trading in the East Indies. Grotius founded his arguments on natural law because, according to him, the notion of the freedom of the seas was essentially a natural law concept.[327] It was also to natural law that Arvid Pardo turned when he sought to propose the concept of common heritage of mankind to the UN General Assembly. According to Pardo, from natural law one could derive an ethic of responsible stewardship of the resources of the deep seabed and ocean floor in the interests of all mankind. Likewise, and for the same interests of mankind, today we are proposing that the human genome be made the common heritage of mankind because, as explained earlier, the patent system is not conducive to the responsible exploitation of the human genome. In our endeavour to do so, there are lessons to be learnt from both Grotius and Pardo. From Grotius we learn that nature has given 'all things' to 'all people'[328] and from this he finds justification for the law of prize and the natural right to trade which must therefore comport the right of free passage. From Pardo we learn that the concept of common heritage of mankind can be the new model of property management for the international community as fulfilment of the stewardship obligations derived from natural law. In other words, while natural law

---

[326] Rimmer, *Intellectual Property and Biotechnology*, pp. 188–89.

[327] Esther D. Reed, 'Property Rights, Genes and Common Good', *Journal of Religious Ethics*, 34:1 (2006), 41–67.

[328] Hugo Grotius, *Freedom of the Seas: The Right of the Dutch to Take Part in the East Indian Trade*, trans. by Ralph Van Deman Magoffin (New York: Oxford University, 1966), p. 14. <http://www.oll.libertyfund.org/EBOOKS/Grotius_0049.pdf> [accessed on 22 August 2006]

explains the genesis of the stewardship model as a moral obligation, the concept of common heritage of mankind provides a suitable political regime for the management of these resources in the interests of all mankind.

It is easy to find a parallel between the situation faced by Grotius in dealing with the Spanish and Portuguese claims to exclude foreigners from navigating or entering their waters and the problems faced by all those involved in the biomedical field as a result of the emerging anti-commons effect on biomedical research generated by the immense proliferation of patents granted over the past decade on downstream research.[329] Just as Spain sought to ban others from navigating the Pacific Ocean and the Gulf of Mexico while Portugal sought to exclude others from navigating the Atlantic south of Morocco and the Indian Ocean, biotechnology firms are today handicapping biomedical research by acquiring more patents and expanding their scope with more licensing and litigating. The result is the *tragedy of the anti-commons* where resources are being underused because of gatekeeper-patents that bar other researchers from pursuing their work on developing important new healthcare products. Information that was originally placed in the public domain by several genome projects becomes the proprietary research of both public and private companies with other researchers being denied free access to the information and materials necessary to pursue their biological research. So, for example, if the characterization of nucleic acid sequences does not remain freely available, then researchers will be excluded from using these nucleic acids to develop new therapeutics and diagnostics. Basically these territorial claims on biomedical research are being achieved by many companies through acquiring large number of patents for purely defensive reasons so as to avoid having to negotiate with other patent holders.[330] At the moment there appear to be two mechanisms responsible for creating the anti-commons effect, namely (i) by the creation of too many fragments of intellectual property rights in potential future products and (ii) by permitting too many upstream patent holders to stack licenses on top of the future discoveries of downstream users.[331] So, as foreseeable commercial products are likely to use multiple DNA fragments, a proliferation of patents on individual

---

[329]   Deborah Frohriep Pestalozi, *The Case of Anticommons in Biomedical Research* (MAS_IP Diploma Papers & Research Reports), Module 115 'US-Patents' Paper 3 (2006).

[330]   Nikolaus Thumm, 'Patents for Genetic Inventions: A Tool to Promote Technological Advance or a Limitation for Upstream Inventions?', *Technovation*, 25 (2005), 1410–17.

[331]   Resnik, 'A Biotechnology Patent Pool'.

fragments held by different owners will inevitably require costly future transactions to bundle licenses together before a firm can have an effective right to develop these products. The result is that firms may opt to divert their attention to other products that are covered by less licensing obstacles or to proceed to animal and then clinical testing on the basis of incomplete information. An anti-commons can also be created with the use of reach-through license agreements on patented research tools. These patented research tools can give the owner of a patented invention rights in subsequent downstream discoveries that can take the form of royalties or an exclusive or non-exclusive license on future discoveries or an option to acquire a license. The problem with research patented tools is that as upstream owners stack overlapping and inconsistent claims on potential downstream products, they effectively win the right to be continually present at the bargaining table as a research project moves downstream towards product development.[332]

Grotius' purpose in writing *Mare Liberum* was to create some form of regulation and state practice based on the notion that the freedom of the high seas was a natural law concept. Arvid Pardo sought to protect and regulate, by means of an international authority, the resources of the deep seabed. Today politicians, legal theorists and moralists are agonizing over issues surrounding the human genome which has proved one of those complex challenges that Pardo foresaw way back in 1968 when he first proposed the concept of common heritage of mankind to the First Committee of the General Assembly of the United Nations:

> It is a new legal principle that we wish to introduce into international law, it is a legal principle which, we feel, must receive recognition if the international community is to cope constructively and effectively with the ever more complex challenges which will confront us in the coming decades.[333]

It is not enough that the human genome was declared the common heritage of mankind by the UNESCO in 1997. Nor is it particularly significant that the US President Bill Clinton and the British Prime Minister Tony Blair, in their Joint Statement of 14 March 2000, agreed that there should be open access to the human genome sequence. This statement was nothing more than an echo of the statement that US President Lyndon Johnson had made in 1966 to the effect that

---

[332]   Heller and Eisenberg, 'Can Patents Deter Innovation', pp. 698–701.

[333]   Pardo, *The Common Heritage of Mankind*, p. 64.

the deep seas and the ocean bottom were the legacy of all human beings[334] which meant that they were open to exploitation by all those nations who had the means to do so. Likewise the Clinton-Blair statement, while lauding on the one hand, the rapid progress being made in human genome research and its contribution towards finding effective treatments, preventions and cures, it deliberately refrained from proclaiming the human genome the common heritage of mankind because there was never any intention on the part of the two political leaders to do so—in a nutshell, the Joint Statement was more of a political slogan than a genuine nod in the direction of making the human genome the common heritage of mankind. I would dare add that Clinton and Blair, like the majority of other political leaders and legal theorists and economists who have written on the common heritage of mankind, have not fathomed the radical nature of the concept. At the same time, the squabbling between the developed countries and less developed countries during the proceedings of the Law of the Sea Convention produced a travesty of the Pardosian concept of the common heritage of mankind.

There will never be a better time than now to apply the concept of common heritage of mankind to the human genome by restoring to the concept its philosophical birthright. This has sadly been hitherto, for the greater part, totally ignored in the controversial debates that the concept has generated since the Maltese Government, on 17 August 1967, asked the Secretary-General of the UN to include a Supplementary Item in the Agenda of the 22nd Session of the UN General Assembly with the title, Declaration and Treaty Concerning the Reservation Exclusively for Peaceful Purposes of the Seabed and of the Ocean Floor, Underlying the Seas Beyond the Limits of Present National Jurisdiction, and the Use of their Resources in the Interests of Mankind.[335] The request was accepted and on 1 November 1967, Arvid Pardo embarked on a long and learned disposition in which he gave birth to the concept of common heritage of mankind amidst the wonders of the deep seabed.[336] In our endeavour to make the human genome the common heritage of mankind, Pardo's exposition of the common

---

[334]   Address given by President Lyndon Johnson at the commissioning of the vessel, *U.S. NOAA Oceanographer*, 13 July 1966.

[335]   Arvid Pardo, Note Verbale to the Secretary-General, 22nd Sess., Annex, Mem., UN Doc. A/6695 (17 August 1967) (Request for the Inclusion of a Supplementary Item in the Agenda of the Twenty-Second Session).

[336]   Yuwen Li, *Transfer of Technology for Deep Sea-Bed Mining: The 1982 Law of the Sea Convention and Beyond* (Dordrecht: Martinus Nijhoff Publishers, 1994), p. 17.

heritage concept remains the foundational source of our philosophical thinking on the human genome.

2.3 The Birthright of the Common Heritage of Mankind

As stated earlier, the sources which have given rise to the concept of common heritage of mankind are natural law and the ethic of stewardship which Arvid Pardo put in a suitable jacket of international management for the benefit of all mankind. So it is fair to say that when Pardo stood up to address the General Assembly on 1 November 1967, he was not so much introducing a new moral political innovation as reiterating a universal and intertemporal moral principle derived from natural law which holds that the existence of moral and legal principles must derive their validity and authority from the natural conditions of human existence, the natural order of the universe or the eternal law of God. The philosophical underpinnings of the concept of common heritage of mankind apply equally to the natural resources of the deep seabed and ocean floor as to the human genome.

Natural law refers specifically to the tradition of moral, political and legal thinking which has developed, particularly within Catholicism, since the time of Aquinas and which regards his ethical and political writings as the classical source. As a moral theory, it emphasizes the role of reason or *Recta Ratio* in our moral deliberations:

> One ought to keep in mind that the nature of each and every thing is chiefly determined by the form whereby it is specified. Man is specified by his rational soul, properly speaking, and therefore anything contrary to the order of reason is contrary to the nature of man as such...Accordingly, human virtue, which makes both man himself and his work good, is in accord with human nature only to the extent that it is in accord with reason; and vice is contrary to human nature to the extent that it is contrary to the order of reason.[337]

For Aquinas, natural law is 'an ordinance of reason for the common good made by the authority who has care of the community and promulgated'.[338] This authority, to Aquinas, is God who promulgates natural law by 'instilling it into men's minds that they can know it because of what they really are'.[339]

---

[337] St. Thomas Aquinas, *Summa Theologiae: Sin*, ed. /trans. by John Fearon O.P., 60 vols (London: Blackfriars, 1975), XXV, p. 9. (ST, Ia2ae, q. 71, a.2).

[338] St. Thomas Aquinas, *Summa Theologiae: Law and Political Theory*, ed. /trans. by Thomas Gilby O.P., 60 vols (London: Blackfriars, 1975), XXVIII, p. 17. (ST, 1ae2ae, q. 90, a.4).

[339] Ibid.

Hence, *Recta Ratio* was that function of man that distinguished him from all other creatures and as a practical principle, 'it harmonized the various ends appropriate to the different spheres of individual and group existence'.[340] It follows that the natural law doctrine of ownership can provide the philosophical framework for the moral evaluation of contemporary economic arrangements including the ownership of the world's natural resources. As a matter of act, natural law discussions of property since Aquinas have always sought to elaborate a set of moral standards by which decisions of owners and established ownership arrangements could be morally evaluated and the development of better arrangements rationally guided. Three self-evident but underived natural law precepts may be inferred, namely (i) the preservation of mankind, (ii) the preservation of society and (iii) the worship of God.[341]

Aquinas sees man's exercise of natural dominion from a purely theological perspective where it is God who has made the earth and man is given dominion over it in virtue of his intellectual nature:

> We can consider external things in two ways. Looked at first of all from the point of view of their nature, this is not subject to man's power, but only to God's sovereign power. Alternatively, they can be looked at from the point of view of their use and management, and in this regard man has a natural dominion over external things, for he has a mind and a will with which to turn them to his account'.[342]

According to Andrew Lustig, several implications follow from this assertion, chief among them that the goods of the earth, including natural resources, initially belonged to all of mankind and not, as such, to individual owners. Again, the nature of property is essentially social in nature because access to the goods of the earth was primarily established in terms of common use and not private ownership.[343]

So for Aquinas, while it is natural for humans to have dominion over the world of nature, this does not mean that they own the world of nature. He refers to man's dominion or use over 'exterior things', 'other creatures' or 'inferior

---

[340]   B. Andrew Lustig, 'Natural Law, Property and Justice: The General Justification of Property in John Locke', in *Thomas Aquinas*, ed. by John Inglis (Aldershot: Ashgate, 2006), p. 292.

[341]   St. Thomas Aquinas, *Summa Theologiae: Law and Political Theory*, ed. /trans. by Thomas Gilby O.P., 60 vols. (London: Blackfriars, 1975), XXVIII, pp. 77–83. (ST, Ia2ae, q.94, a.2).

[342]   St. Thomas Aquinas, *Summa Theologiae: Injustice*, ed./trans. by Marcus Lefebure O.P., 60 vols. (London: Blackfriars, 1975), XXXVIII, p. 65. (ST, 2a2ae, q.66, a.1).

[343]   Lustig, *Natural Law*, p. 293.

creatures'[344] as possession but by this, he does not mean that the things used by man are subject to appropriation by any individual or group:

> God has pre-eminent dominion over all things, and in his providence he ordered certain things for men's material support. This is why it is natural for man to have dominion over things in the sense of having power to use them.[345]

In Aquinas' eyes, this kind of possession is synonymous with 'holding things in common'. The distinction between 'having things in common' and 'private ownership' is understandable given the theological context in which Aquinas sought to elaborate moral standards related to issues of ownership. Implicit in his natural law conception of ownership were mainly three things, namely (i) that man was a rational being, (ii) that he had possession over other creatures and most importantly, (iii) that his dominion over the world of nature did not infringe on the prerogatives of either God or nature itself. It follows that for Aquinas, man is morally justified in exercising dominion over the world of nature, including the world's natural resources as long as this relation of dominion is understood as 'having things in common' rather than 'private ownership'.

Man can possess something as his own (*quasi propriam*) and show no concern for others' needs or man can take care of and dispose of things (*potestas procurandi et dispensandi*) with discretion and so, in his use of things, he allows himself to be guided by the requirements of the common good. Aquinas maintains that natural justice demands that the use of exterior things such as the world's natural resources should be common rather than private.

Although natural justice demands that all persons are treated with the same respect, it is not to be excluded that some individuals may be treated differently on the basis of dessert or need as long as such different treatment does not, in any way, discriminate against any other person. This distinction is related to the use of exterior things discussed above in the sense that although it is a fundamental requirement of the common good that all things are held in common, sometimes the common good is best served when some exterior things are appropriated by some individuals or groups and not held in common. Usually

---

[344] St. Thomas Aquinas, *Summa Theologiae: Injustice*, ed./trans. by Marcus Lefebure O.P., 60 vols. (London: Blackfriars, 1975), XXXVIII, pp. 63–65. (ST, 2a2ae, q.66,a.1).

[345] When Thomas Aquinas talks about dominion over 'other creatures' or 'inferior creatures' he was not aware of the environmental problems that we are faced with today. He was more inclined towards 'dominating' nature rather than 'conforming' to nature but he had no idea of the extremes to which 'domination' of nature would be taken.

things are better taken care of when they fall under the responsibility of identifiable individuals or groups than when they are left in the hands of everyone. This kind of arrangement is more conducive towards governing society in an orderly fashion and discourages those conflicts which are bound to take place when people hold things in common without division:

> Man has a twofold competence in relation to material things. The first is the title to care for and distribute the earth's resources. Understood in this way, it is not merely legitimate for a man to possess things as his own, it is even necessary for human life and this for three reasons. First, because each person takes more trouble to care for something that is his sole responsibility than what is held in common or by many—for in such a case each individual shirks the work and leaves the responsibility to somebody else, which is what happens when too many officials are involved. Second, because human affairs are more efficiently organized if each person has his own responsibility to discharge; and there would be chaos if everybody cared for everything. Third because men live together in greater peace where everyone is content with his task. We do, in fact, notice that quarrels often break out amongst men who hold things in common without distinction.[346]

So for Aquinas, although ideally, property should be held in common, private property may be permitted. In a sense, private property is justified in the service of the common good! His view of private property is clearly very different from that of the earlier Roman law of property that gave the owner the power to use and misuse (*jus utendi et abutendi*). Private property, for Aquinas remains subject to the natural law moral precept that in times of need, all property must be considered common. This is *dominium utile* as opposed to the classical notion of absolute *dominium* with no reference to social need.

In synthesis, private property, for Aquinas, is a relative and not an absolute right. It is a good way of ensuring a peaceful society and generally a good way of managing the goods of the earth. He does not approve of ownership for the sake of ownership—man should not treat the goods of the earth as solely his but as if they were common. This is essentially the idea of stewardship where ownership is not seen as absolute dominion but responsible management of the goods of the earth for the benefit of all mankind. Applied to the world's natural resources, the requirement of common use would demand that there be an international political authority capable of regulating the exploitation of the world's natural resources in the interests of all mankind.[347]

---

[346]   St. Thomas Aquinas, *Summa Theologiae: Injustice*, ed./trans. by Marcus Lefebure O.P., 60 vols. (London: Blackfriars, 1975), XXXVIII, pp. 67–69. (ST, 2a2ae, q.66,a.2).

[347]   Joseph Boyle, 'Natural Law, Ownership and the World's Natural Resources', in *Thomas Aquinas*, ed. by John Inglis (Aldershot: Ashgate, 2006), p. 203.

The moral implications derived from traditional natural law theory are that there are certain basic principles and obligations that bind all states and the international community as a whole, equally and unconditionally. Once it is made clear that the common heritage of mankind is a necessary extension of natural law theory, it follows that the provisions of the concept need only be enunciated since they always belonged to mankind!

2.4 The Common Heritage of Mankind as a Model of Political Stewardship

As explained earlier, the sources which have fed the concept of common heritage of mankind are natural law and the ethic of stewardship. The stewardship theology is to be found in all major religious traditions, namely the Judeo-Christian, Islamic and Buddhist traditions. In these religions, human beings are seen as trustees of God who have responsibilities not only for other creatures but also for future generations. This is a human-centred ethic that is based on human choices rather than choices within the domain of other species—human beings are not one species among many but *the species* entrusted with the responsibility to care for all other species. Human beings are entrusted with such a task because they are able to exercise dominion in virtue of their intellectual nature which is able to discern the fundamental truths that form the basis of natural law, namely the preservation of mankind and society and the worship of God. According to Paul Ramsey, the right of property is to be understood as the stewardship of property which can never condone dominion, private or otherwise:

> Stewardship means that a thing may be ours in that we are persons in covenant, and that property should be held and used in fealty toward God and in recognition of His Sovereign right and sole dominion and, indivisible from this, it should be held and used in fealty of life with our fellow men.[348]

Today the ethic of stewardship can be understood as the responsible use of natural resources in a way that takes full and balanced account of the interests of

---

[348] William Werpehowski and Stephen D. Crocco (eds.), *The Essential Paul Ramsey: A Collection* (New Haven: Yale University Press, 1994), p. 116.

society, future generations and other species as well as of private needs and accepts significant answerability to society.[349] Given this philosophical perspective, the stewardship ethic, which can have both secular and religious interpretations, can form the basis of a public trust doctrine for the sharing of the benefits, among all mankind, of the natural resources of the planet such as the bounties of the deep sea bed or the fruits of genomic research. The ethical aspects of stewardship provide an explicit, rational and moral underpinning for our treatment of natural resources, the human genome and the natural world and challenge other forms of management or exploitation of resources, particularly those based on indifference to the natural world, human greed, expediency or fashion.[350]

The stewardship metaphor needs clarification in two aspects, namely the question of dominion and management. The idea of dominion given by God to man over other creatures may appear, as a result of a misreading of the metaphorical meaning of stewardship, to justify an exploitative relation of man versus nature.[351] This interpretation may also be suggested by the natural law theory of Aquinas where man again appears to be morally justified in exercising dominion over the world of nature in virtue of his rational nature. These interpretations are wrong because they fail to explain the implications of duties to care for the rest of creation that are inherent in both natural law theory and the stewardship ethic. For the Muslim, for example, mankind's role on earth is that of a *Khalifah* or trustee of *Allah*:

> We are Allah's stewards and agents on Earth. We are not masters of this Earth; it does not belong to us to do what we wish. It belongs to Allah and he has entrusted us with its safekeeping. Our function as viceregents, Khalifahs of Allah, is only to oversee the trust.[352]

So, as steward on earth, mankind is charged with the protection and preservation of the environment which entails using natural resources without undue

---

[349]   Richard Worrell and Michael C. Appleby, 'Stewardship of Natural Resources: Definition, Ethical and Practical Aspects', *Journal of Agricultural and Environmental Ethics,* 12 (2000), 263–77.

[350]   Ibid., p. 266.

[351]   Lynn White, 'The Historical Roots of our Ecological Crisis', *Science,* 155 (1967), 1203–07.

[352]   Abdullah Omar Nasif, 'The Muslim Declaration of Nature', *Environmental Policy and Law,* 17:1 (1987), 47.

waste.[353] At the same time, the stewardship model does not tell us *how* to use these resources! It explains a moral obligation but it does not provide a political structure. Pardo filled this lacuna in the stewardship model with his proposal for a legal regime that would be responsible for the international management of the common heritage by and for mankind.

The stewardship model is also radically different from the sustainable management model concept of *common concern of mankind* (CCM) that was first used in the UN General Assembly Resolution 43/53 of 1988.[354] The basic difference between the two concepts was that whereas the stewardship model that is at the root of the common heritage of mankind as proposed by Pardo was founded on the concept of 'non-appropriation',[355] the concept of *common concern of mankind* was totally free from such non-appropriation connotations. According to Kirgis, the concept of *common concern of mankind* was used in order to avoid the political ramifications of the concept of common heritage of mankind that was still being debated in the context of the deep seabed and outer space.[356]

The focus of the UN Resolution in favour of Climate Change was to bind states to maintain a minimum of environmental protection, to fulfill their legal obligations concerning the global environment and to authorize the international community to employ the necessary means to ensure the protection of those natural resources that are considered the *common concern of mankind*.[357] The Joint Statement of US President Bill Clinton and UK Prime Minister Tony Blair of 14 March 2000 in which they said that 'raw fundamental data on the human genome, including the human DNA sequence and its variations, should be made freely available to scientists everywhere' was more an expression of the human

---

[353] Abdul Wahid Hamid, *Islam: The Natural Way*, quoted in Baslar, *The Concept of Common Heritage of Mankind in International Law*, p. 15.

[354] UNGA Res. 43/53 on the Protection of Global Climate for Present and Future Generations of Mankind, adopted on 6 December 1988.

[355] Pardo, *The Common Heritage of Mankind*, pp. 41–42.

[356] F. L. Kirgis, 'Standing Challenge Human Endeavours that Could Change the Climate', *American Journal of International Law*, 84:2 (1990), 525–30 (p. 525). See also, F. Biermann, 'Saving the Atmosphere: International Law, Developing Countries and Air Pollution', *European Journal of International Law*, 10:3 (1999), 549–82.

[357] UNGA Res. 43/53 on the Protection of Global Climate for Present and Future Generations of Mankind, adopted on 6 December 1988.

genome as a *common concern of mankind* rather than an affirmation of the human genome as common heritage of mankind.[358] Taking into consideration the part of the Statement just quoted and the fact that, as already mentioned in our study, the USPTO reiterated, within a week of the Joint Statement, that the leaders' words did not in any way affect the patenting system, it becomes very clear that their intention was only to make the human genome a *common concern of mankind* because the appropriation of the human genome through the patenting system was never called into question!

The Roman Catholic Church has always been a staunch supporter of the concept of common heritage of mankind and the stewardship model of management of the world's natural resources. Already in 1931 Pope Pius XI had made the important distinction between the 'right to own property' and the 'right to use property', arguing that the State may, in the interests of the common good, limit the use of private property.[359] This fundamental distinction is at the basis of the concept of common heritage of mankind and the stewardship model of resource management. When Arvid Pardo addressed the UN General Assembly in 1967, this distinction between the 'right to own' and the 'right to use' was the key to making the resources of the deep seabed and ocean floor the common heritage of mankind to be managed for the good of all humanity.[360] But more importantly, the stewardship model of management, which for Pardo was at the basis of the concept of common heritage of mankind, incorporated the proviso, already contemplated by Pope Pius XI, that in the interests of all mankind, the 'right to use' may also be limited. To Pardo this meant, in no uncertain terms, that the US and other industrialized countries would have to relinquish their right to exploit the resources of the deep seabed and ocean floor, even though they had the potential to develop the technology necessary to do so. The same situation may prevail in the near future when, in order to combat the *tragedy of the anti-commons*, public and private pharmaceutical companies may be called upon to relinquish broad patents, just to give one example, that are hindering downstream biomedical research.

---

[358] Bill Clinton and Tony Blair, Joint Statement by President William Clinton and Prime Minister Tony Blair of the United Kingdom (14 March 2000) <http://wwwipmall.info/hosted_resources/ippresdocs/ippd_44.htm, 14 March> [accessed on 20 March 2006]

[359] Pope Pius XI, *Quaragesimo Anno*, 1931. <http://www.vatican.va/holy_father/pius_xi/encyclicals/documents/hf_p-xi_enc_19310515_quadragesimo-anno_en.html> [accessed on 15 September 2007]

[360] Borgese, *Pacem in Maribus*, pp. 161–62.

Then in 1963, the unexpected encyclical *Pacem in Terris* of Pope John XXIII was published with social and political reverberations that took the world by surprise. In the encyclical, John XXIII writes about the common good and anticipates the kind of world ethic that Arvid Pardo thought necessary if the concept of common heritage of mankind was to make a difference on the world scene:

> In the second place, the very nature of the common good requires that all members of the state be entitled to share in it, although in different ways according to each one's tasks, merits and circumstances. For this reason, every civil authority must take pains to promote the common good of all, without preference for any single citizen or civic group. As Our Predecessor of immortal memory, Leo XIII, has said: 'The civil power must not serve the advantage of any one individual, or some few persons, inasmuch as it was established for the common good of all'. Considerations of justice and equity, however, can at times demand that those involved in civil government give more attention to the less fortunate members of the community, since they are less able to defend their rights and to assert their legitimate claims.[361]

With the encyclical, Pope John wanted to advise world leaders that as the world was becoming increasingly interdependent and global, the common good of humanity could only be achieved if there was international cooperation. For Pope John XXIII, a universal common good could only be advanced by an international authority, established by the consent of nations rather than by coercion. It is the same kind of international authority that Pardo envisaged for the management of the resources of the deep seabed and ocean floor and that we will be proposing in the course of this research, for the management of the human genome.

Reiterating the position of the Roman Catholic Church's stewardship ethic in his encyclical *De Populorum Progressio* of 1967, Pope Paul VI wrote:

> God intended the Earth and all that it contains for the use of every human being and people. Thus all men follow justice and unite in charity; created goods should abound for them on reasonable basis.[362]

---

[361] Pope John XXIII – *Pacem in Terris*, 1963. <http://www.vatican.va/holy_father/john_xxiii/encyclicals/documents/hf_j-xxiii_enc_11041963_pacem_en.html> [accessed on 15 September 2007]

[362] Pope Paul VI – *De Populorum Progressio*, 1967. <http://www.vatican.va/holy_father/paul_vi/encyclicals/documents/hf_p-vi_enc_26031967_populorum_en.html> [accessed on 15 September 2007]

Again, in his message to the 1972 Stockholm Conference Pope Paul VI insisted that:

> No one can take possession in an absolute and specific way of the environment, which is not a *res nullius*—something not belonging to anyone—but a *res omnium*—the patrimony of mankind; consequently those possessing it—privately and publicly—must use it in a way that rebounds to everyone's advantage.[363]

Paul VI's words are an echo of Arvid Pardo's admonition that if we do not assume the responsible stewardship of the resources of the deep seabed and ocean floor by making them the common heritage of mankind, we are incurring the risk of losing these resources to the handful of developed countries that have the necessary technology to explore and extract them.[364] As already explained, the *laissez faire laissez passer* attitude of the high seas permitted such an unjust and inequitable distribution of the resources of the deep seabed!

2.5   The Common Heritage of Mankind as a Challenge to Legal Positivism

It was Hugo Grotius who transposed the basic elements of Aquinas' natural law to the secular realm. As a matter of fact, Grotius is considered to be the first natural law theorist to separate natural law as a creation of reason from its theological context.[365] The basis of the distinction between the two branches of natural law theory, one theological and the other secular has its origin in the belief, common in both ancient and medieval accounts of the theory, that although the law of nature was implanted in man by God, belief in God was not an essential part of the theory because this law was the law of our nature—a belief implicitly affirmed by Aquinas when he distinguished between the natural law and the eternal law of God.[366]

The fundamental principles of natural law are stated very clearly in the writings of Grotius who stood in the broad tradition of natural law theory in

---

363   Emmanuel Agius and Lionel Chircop, *Caring for Future Generations: Jewish, Christian and Islamic Perspectives* (Westport, Conn: Praeger, 1998), p. 105.

364   Pardo, *The Common Heritage of Mankind*, p. 90.

365   Ernest Bloch, *Natural Law and Human Dignity*, quoted in Reed, 'Property Rights, Genes and Common Good', pp. 41–67 (p. 42).

366   Stephen Buckle, 'Natural Law', in *A Companion to Ethics*, ed. by Peter Singer (Oxford: Blackwell Publishers, 1993) p. 167.

which it was assumed that positive law, including the rights and obligations of property, should be rooted in the law of nature. After Grotius, the development of modern natural law became markedly detached from the Christian doctrine of the law of nature implanted in humans and revealed by God and more associated with secularist rationalism. Grotius is also lauded as the father of international law as he formulated fundamental principles that have since shaped ideas of international society and the practice of inter-state relations.[367] In his major work, *On the Law of War and Peace*,[368] Grotius adjudicates in detail on the common sources of dispute that lead nations into conflict. His hope was to provide a moral framework for nations that could thereby serve to secure peace. In the *Prolegomena* and opening chapter of the book, he gives a brief account of the general principles that should govern such an enquiry and this list provides the basis of modern natural law.[369]

After the Second World War, the institutional architecture of international society changed enormously. Having gone through the ordeal of a world war, people became passionately aware of the need to protect human rights and natural rights in the interests of all humanity. So on 26 June 1945 the Charter of the United Nations was signed in San Francisco to be followed, in the same year, with the establishment of the World Bank and the International Monetary Fund after the Bretton Woods Conference between the Allied powers in 1944. Another significant event in this emerging political scenario concerned with humanitarian issues was the establishment of the International Military Tribunal for the Punishment of War Criminals in 1945.

Many writers traced the roots of the post-war concern for humanitarian and environmental issues to a modernized version of natural law which was grounded in the dignity of man rather than in the law of God. It was the politico-economic situation of the post-war period that led to the emergence of this new formulation of natural law in accordance with the ultimate benefit of mankind.[370]

---

[367]   Hedley Bull, 'The Importance of Grotius in the Study of International Relations', in *Hugo Grotius and International Relations*, ed. by Benedict Kingsbury, Hedley Bull and Adam Roberts (Oxford: Clarendon Press, 1990), pp. 65–80.

[368]   Hugo Grotius, *On the Law of War and Peace*, trans. by A.C. Campbell (London 1814). <http://www.constitution.org/gro/djbp.htm> [accessed on 22 August 2006]

[369]   Buckle, 'Natural Law', pp. 166–67.

[370]   Baslar, *Common Heritage*, p. 21.

N. Singh[371] sees the invisible hand of natural law in the fundamental rights of mankind in the preamble to the UN Charter[372] and in the first and second-generation rights to peace and life that were enshrined in the UN Declaration of Human Rights.[373] He sees the same natural law influence behind the third-generation rights to an adequate environment and to sustainable development that were proclaimed in the Stockholm Declaration of 1972[374] and the Rio Declaration of 1992.[375]

M.V. White argues that the 'common heritage of mankind embodies the spirit of an emerging world economic order based on egalitarian principles'. He also sees the common heritage of mankind as,

> ...a philosophical and legal tool which can be useful for equitable distribution of the world's wealth as well as a basis for global sharing of scarce resources.[376]

Even on an institutional level there is evident a departure from a state-centric international system to a human-centric law of mankind. The wordings of the 1972 Stockholm Declaration, the 1982 World Charter for Nature[377] and the 1992 Rio Declaration, all attest to this when they call upon the international community to transcend the doctrine of sovereignty, based on legal positivism, in favour of a broader understanding of law that is more suited to satisfy the political and ethical needs of today's international community. Contemporary natural law theorists believe that such a legal substratum can be obtained by an ontological theory of natural law that can resolve many of the legal inadequacies of positive law.[378]

---

[371]   N. Singh, 'Right to Environment and Sustainable Development as a Principle of International Law', in *Studia Diplomatica,* 41:1 (1988), 45–61 (p. 46).

[372]   Charter of the United Nations, signed in San Francisco on 26 June 1945, at the conclusion of the United Nations Conference on International Organization.

[373]   Universal Declaration of Human Rights, adopted by the General Assembly of the United Nations at its 3rd Session on 10 December 1948. UNGA Res. 217 A (III)

[374]   Declaration of the United Nations Conference on the Human Environment, proclaimed in Stockholm, on 16 June 1972.

[375]   Rio Declaration on Environment and Development, proclaimed at the conclusion of the United Nations Conference on Environment and Development in Rio de Janeiro, on 14 June 1992.

[376]   M.V. White, 'The Common Heritage of Mankind Principle: An Assessment', *Case Western Reserve Journal of International Law,* 14 (1982), p. 509.

[377]   World Charter for Nature, adopted by the General Assembly of the United Nations at its 37th Session on 28 October 1982. UNGA Res. 37/7.

[378]   Roger Cotterrell, *The Politics of Jurisprudence* (London: Butterworths, 1989), p. 145.

Eurocentrism and the public law of Europe are the product of the rise of positivist philosophy in the political and legal thought of the eighteenth century and are characterized by three *malaises* that permeate the system and are, *prima facie*, in contradiction with the concept of common heritage of mankind. These three *malaises* are (i) individualism, (ii) nationalism and, (iii) materialism. They reflect the changes that took place in the composition of international society that accompanied other changes in its institutional architecture. Throughout the 1940s and the 1950s, many former colonies acquired their independence and became sovereign members of the United Nations, with UN membership increasing from 51 in 1945 to 99 in 1960.

The concept of common heritage of mankind was, in many ways, the antithesis of these Western principles for a number of reasons. Kemal Baslar[379] argues that, first of all, 'aggressive individualism' resulted in the distribution of territories among numerous states of the world and acquisition of territory was legitimized by claims of sovereignty. So, while sovereignty, on the one hand, is a manifestation of clearly demarcated individual entities, on the other hand, the common heritage of mankind idea preaches the unity of mankind and strong international solidarity. Secondly, while nationalism is reflected in international law in the form of the notion of independence of nation-states and sovereign equality, the common heritage of mankind transcends national boundaries and unites all peoples under the flag of universalism since it is the result of the ecological and economic interdependence of the members of the world community. Addressing the Council of Europe on 3 December 1970, Arvid Pardo had stated:

> Traditionally, international law has been essentially concerned with the regulation of relations between states. In ocean space, however, the time has come to recognize as a basic principle of international law the overriding common interest of mankind in the preservation of the quality of marine environment and in the rational and equitable development of its resources lying beyond national jurisdiction.[380]

So, as the application of the common heritage of mankind necessitated strong supranational authority, it transcended nation-states and threatened their sovereign rights. Therefore, positivism proved to be the most important obstacle to an effective international environmental law, of which the common heritage of mankind is an important part, because positivism created a legal system that has

---

[379] Baslar, *Common Heritage*, pp. 23–29.
[380] Alexander Kiss, 'The Common Heritage of Mankind: Utopia or Reality?', *Law of the Sea*, ed. by Hugo Caminos (Aldershot, Hants: Ashgate/Dartmouth, 2001), p. 324.

traditionally been geared towards self-interest through a *laissez-faire* approach. As Erkki Holmila points out, the crux of the problem for most Western states is that they are not used to being told what to do by the international community. In other words, they are not ready to play the part of good Samaritans by refraining from making use of the riches of the seabed as they wished so as to allow poorer countries who very often do not have the capability to exploit the seabed resources, to have their own share of these seabed resources.[381]

Thirdly, 'technocratic positivism' or 'scientific materialism' accompanied technological innovation, and colonialism established an international system based on mercantilism and capitalism. So, it is fair to say that the 'logical formal rationality of the Western European Legal Structure, writ large, had an economic analogue, namely, capitalism'.[382] As the overriding concern of technocratic positivism was the pursuit of progress at all costs, the ideological clash between this predominantly materialistic concept and the more philosophically inclined concept of common heritage of mankind was inevitable. The concept of common heritage of mankind stands for sustainable management of natural resources on behalf of all humanity and so precludes the notion of unimpeded progress in favour of an ethic of protection, caring and sharing of natural resources for future generations.[383]

This was the spirit behind the formation of the Group of 77[384] in 1963 in an effort to consolidate and thereby strengthen the negotiating power of the developing countries.[385] But more importantly, following an action plan by the G-77, in May 1974 the UN General Assembly adopted the Declaration and Action Programme on the Establishment of a New International Economic Order (NIEO) with the aim of giving developing countries a greater say in how the

---

[381]   Erkki Holmila, 'Common Heritage of Mankind in the Law of the Sea', in *Acta Societatis Martensis*, 1 (2005), 187–205 (p. 189).

[382]   Christopher R. Rossi, *Equity and International Law? A Legal Realist Approach to the Process of International Decision Making*, quoted in Baslar, *The Concept of the Common Heritage of Mankind in International Law* , p. 25.

[383]   Baslar, *Common Heritage*, pp. 25–26.

[384]   The group of 77 is an international organization established in 1966 by 77 developing countries, by a Joint Declaration of the 77 Countries at the first session of the UNCTAD in Geneva. Currently it has 133 members but the name has been retained for historical reasons. <http://www.g77.org/main/main.htm> [accessed on 15 July 2007]

[385]   Arvid Pardo and Elizabeth Mann Borgese, *The New International Economic Order and the Law of the Sea: A Projection*, IOI Occasional Papers No. 4 (Malta: International Ocean Institute, 1975), p. 12.

international system was run in terms of financial and trade matters.[386] This way they would also benefit from the system to a greater extent than they had previously done, including the possibility of a greater degree of redistribution of resources.

For Joynor, the creation of an NIEO gave a new philosophical and legal impetus to the concept of common heritage of mankind.[387] In fact many developing countries considered the concept to be an important pillar to the NIEO.[388] In this 'New World Order', the world would acquire full legal ownership rights on the area considered to be a common heritage of mankind. The beneficiary of any profits derived from the exploitation of mineral resources from the region would be all mankind with preferential treatment being given, however, to developing countries. In line with the NIEO ideology, which, to many developing countries, was the inspiration behind the concept of common heritage of mankind, an 'Authority' would be established, which would have both legal jurisdictional over the common space region and executive power to act as the self-designated trustee for the international community in the region.[389] Under a common heritage of mankind regime, the world community, through the offices of the 'Authority' that was to be established for the purpose, would be able to use the common space region but without any attendant rights of ownership, possession or sovereign acquisition of title.[390]

The designation 'all mankind' as beneficiary of any profits that may be derived from the exploitation of a common space region is a nod in the direction of considering the interests, needs and aspirations of all mankind as being separate and distinct from those of all states and governments.[391] The use of the term 'mankind' in international law, after the Second World War, is seen by some as being indicative of the demise of the positivist school of law that was mainly state-centred since the Grotius' era to a more anthropocentric-centred notion of

---

[386]   Declaration on the Establishment of a New Economic Order, adopted by the General Assembly of the United Nations at its Sixth Special Session on 1 May 1974. UNGA Res. 3201(S-VI)

[387]   Joynor, 'Legal Implications of the Concept of the Common Heritage of Mankind', pp. 190–99.

[388]   Pardo and Borgese, *New International Economic Order*, pp. 1–19.

[389]   Ibid.

[390]   Joynor suggests that the 'Authority' established should be something like the 'International Seabed Authority' ISA) created for Seabed mining in the 1982 UNCLOS III Convention on the Law of the Sea.

[391]   The term 'mankind' became a popular term in international documents after the Second World War as a result of the increased awareness for human rights. Like the 'stewardship' metaphor, it is a concept that has its origin in the classical tradition of natural law.

international law or, put differently, from the law of nations to the law of mankind.[392] International law could therefore be applied, juridically to all mankind which as a philosophical notion is seen to encompass even those peoples who may belong to non-self-governing territories and therefore are not integrated in those political units customarily designated as 'states'. As Joynor remarks, '...the interests, needs and aspirations of 'all mankind' would appear to be greater than the sum of all states' national interests'.[393]

Focusing on the legal implications of the heritage notion of the concept of common heritage of mankind, Joynor points out that underlying this notion is the assumption that common areas should be looked upon inheritances that are transmitted down to heirs by birthright from one generation to another. He employs Arvid Pardo's idea of a common use and access to a property without common ownership under the control of an international organization. In the *Pacem in Maribus* Seminar of 1970, Pardo had made it clear that he preferred using the term 'heritage' to 'property' because of the genesis of the term 'property' in Roman Law where it implied, among other things, the 'right to use and misuse' or *'jus utendi et abutendi'*.[394] According to Joynor, under a common heritage of mankind regime, a common space would be designated as an international patrimony that is handed on from one generation to another with the attendant rights and obligations that are normally associated with inheritances that are passed on to one's heirs. These duties that are incumbent to a trustee of an inheritance include the responsible management of the common space area in a way that does not compromise the needs and interests of future generations especially with regards to the use, exploitation, development and distribution of the region's resources:

> In legal terms the concept of 'common heritage' would require that serious scrutiny be given to every activity in the area in order to prevent resource waste and to preclude environmental abuse. To fail in the protection, conservation, preservation and prudential management of the region and its resources would breach the trust and legal obligation implicit in responsibly supervising the earth's heritage for mankind in the future.[395]

In a word, the concept of common heritage of mankind should not be based on the image of the exploitative management of nature but rather on the image of

---

[392]   A.A. Cocca, *The Law of Mankind: Ius Inter Gentes Again*, quoted in Baslar, *The Concept of Common Heritage of Mankind in International Law* , p. 71.

[393]   Joynor, 'Legal Implications of the Concept of the Common Heritage of Mankind', p. 195.

[394]   Pardo, *The Common Heritage of Mankind*, p. x.

[395]   Joynor, 'Legal Implications of the Concept of the Common Heritage of Mankind', p. 195.

wise management that is able to use the common good in the interest of all mankind.

2.6 Preventing Another *Mare Liberum*

Many philosophers, politicians and legal theorists are today preoccupied over a number of fundamental issues that revolve round the accessibility to human DNA sequences and the criteria for patentability.[396] They are concerned that the snapping up of patents on genes may not lead to powerful new medicines but, on the contrary, quash biomedical innovation. The problem is that many passages from the Book of Life have already been patented and therefore claimed as private property.[397] The international community faces questions about what may and may not be reduced to the state of private property.

The concept of common heritage of mankind incorporates a number of social and political implications which are relevant to our concerns regarding access to the human genome and patenting practices. The first of these defining principles of the common heritage of mankind notion is that these regions of common space areas do not become subject to appropriation of any kind, public or private, national or corporate.[398] These common space regions would be regarded as regions belonging to no one, excluding the possibility of any one claiming sovereignty to them.[399] Hence any jurisdictional privileges, rights or obligations determined by sovereignty are absent and so no agent of any such authority could issue or enforce commands in these regions. In a nutshell, an international area under a common heritage of mankind regime could not be owned legally in whole or in part by any state or group of states—the area would be administered by the international community.[400]

The issue of private or common ownership was originally raised by Hugo Grotius who debated whether the sea could be reduced to the state of private property or whether it should be common to all. His conclusion was that neither

[396] Federico Lenzerini, 'Biotechnology, Human Dignity and the Human Genome', in *Biotechnology and International Law*, ed. by Francesco Francioni and Tullio Scovazzi (Oxford: Hart Publishing, 2006), pp. 285–340.

[397] Regalado, 'The Great Gene Grab', pp. 49–50.

[398] Arvid Pardo, 'First Statement to the First Committee of the General Assembly 1 November 1967', in *The Common Heritage of Mankind: Selected Papers on Oceans and World Order 1967–1974* (Malta: Malta University Press, 1975), pp. 1–41.

[399] Holmila, 'Common Heritage of Mankind in the Law of the Sea', pp. 195–97.

[400] Joynor, 'Legal Implications of the Concept of the Common Heritage of Mankind', p. 191.

the Spanish nor the Portuguese had rights to prevent the Dutch from sailing to the East Indies and trading. God, he said, would not allow to escape unpunished those, who, 'for the sake of private gain, opposed a common benefit of the human race'.[401] The magnitude of the sea was such as to be 'sufficient for the use of all nations'—all should be allowed, without inconvenience and prejudice to each other, the right to fish, sail and to use the sea for any other advantage they could derive from it.[402]

Arvid Pardo, while sharing Grotius' belief that the sea should not be reduced to a state of private property, was not so sure that the sea was an unfathomable resource, 'sufficient for the use of all nations'. In fact he was deeply concerned that rapidly developing technology would soon make possible the exploration, occupation and exploitation of the world's sea beds and much of the ocean floor. Inevitably this would lead to the appropriation, for national use, of the seabed and ocean floor underlying the seas beyond national jurisdiction with consequences for all countries that may be incalculable.[403]

In our day we are called to use Grotius' arguments in defence of a common ownership of the sea in order to combat against the private appropriation of the human genome and its subsequent commercialization through the granting of exclusive intellectual propriety rights. At the same time, we must prevent another *Mare Liberum* because the human genome is not the limitless resource that Grotius imagined the sea to be—already one-fifth of the human genome is under patent! Here we concur with Arvid Pardo who was concerned with the *laissez faire* attitude that accompanied Grotius' *Mare Liberum*. The human genome presents an equivalent cause for concern considering the unrestrictive patent practices in biomedical research that are creating an anti-commons effect and leading to, paradoxically, fewer new medicines and treatments for the relief of suffering and the improvement of human health.

The second defining characteristic of the common heritage of mankind principle is that under a CHM regime, all people would be expected to share in

---

[401]   Grotius, *Freedom of the Seas.* <http://www.oll.libertyfund.org/EBOOKS/Grotius_0049.pdf> [accessed on 22 August 2006]

[402]   Hugo Grotius, *The Rights of War and Peace*, trans. by A.C. Campbell (New York: M. Walter Dunne, 1901) <http://oll.libertyfund.org/?option=com_staticxt&staticfile=show.php%3Fti-tle=553&chapter=90754&layout=html&Itemid=27> [accessed on 20 February 2006] (Chapter II, para. 3)

[403]   Pardo, *The Common Heritage of Mankind*, p. 2.

the management of a common space area.[404] In other words, states or national governments will be precluded from this legal action save as the representative agents of all mankind. This will ensure that decisions affecting the region will be motivated by universal popular interests rather than national interests.[405]

The third defining characteristic is that if natural resources are exploited from a common space area, any economic benefits derived from such exploitation should be shared internationally such that all of mankind will benefit. Under a CHM regime, agencies engaged in commercial profit or private gain would be deemed inappropriate unless they operated to enhance the common benefit of all mankind. Hence, the manganese nodules on the deep seabed, exotic elements and metals in celestial bodies and possibly hard minerals and hydrocarbons in Antarctica and offshore would fall under the prohibition of non-exploitability, save under the auspices of a common space regime mandate.

In an article appearing in *Science*, Bartha Knoppers has suggested that the Grotian legal theory of *res communis* that argues for 'common use' as opposed to 'private use' of property has considerable relevance to the contemporary debate on genetic benefit sharing in that it creates an international precedent that can be employed to argue in favour of regarding the human genome as a 'common heritage'.[406] She believes that the precedent created by Grotius in the context of the navigation of the high seas is particularly illuminating in the present political situation that sees modern liberal concepts of individual autonomy and private property obstructing attempts to elaborate an adequate ethic of law and genetics to meet present-day needs.[407] According to Knoppers, Grotius' law of the sea of the seventeenth century together with international law governing air and space of the twentieth century set the stage for making the human genome a 'common heritage'.[408]

---

[404]   Ryuichi, 'Human Genome as Common Heritage of Mankind Proposal'. <http://www.eubios.info/ASIAE/BIAE59.htm> [accessed on 28 January 2000]

[405]   Holmila, 'Common Heritage of Mankind in the Law of the Sea', pp. 198–200.

[406]   Bartha Maria Knoppers, 'Genetic Benefit Sharing', *Science*, 290:6 (2000), 49.

[407]   Esther D. Reed, 'Property Rights, Genes, and Common Good', *Journal of Religious Ethics*, 34:1 (2006), 41–67 (p. 53).

[408]   Bartha Maria Knoppers, 'The Human Genome: Individual Property or Common Heritage', in *The Human Genome*, co-ord. by Jean-Francois Mattei (Strasbourg: Council of Europe Publishing, 2006), pp. 109–16.

Initial attempts to prevent another *Mare Liberum* with the human genome were taken by the International Federation of Gynaecology and Obstetrics Committee for the Study of Ethical Aspects of Human Reproduction when, in its study entitled *Patenting of Human Genes*,[409] it noted that if the human genome is seen by many as belonging to everyone, then allowing the privatization of certain genes was tantamount to a 'private take-over of our common heritage'. Although the Committee was uneasy with the language of private ownership, it was unable to come up with an alternative concept or language in its place. Progress was made by The Human Genome Organization (HUGO) Ethics Committee when on 9 April 2000, it released a statement introducing the concepts of 'common heritage' and 'benefit sharing'.[410] The statement's objective was to advance the concept of benefit sharing with a view to directing research and profit-making entities towards the fostering of health for all human beings.

2.7   Making the Common Heritage of Mankind a Legal Principle of International Law

The purpose of this study is to make the human genome the common heritage of mankind. Lessons can be learnt from the UN Law of the Sea Convention (UNCLOS) where the common heritage of mankind was applied to the resources of the deep seabed and ocean floor after a tumultuous twenty-five years of negotiations. The end result was the first in international law with the establishment of a regime for the management of resources by an international organization. In the next section of our study, we will follow the path taken to transform the common heritage of mankind from a philosophical concept to a legal principle of international law. At the same time, we will be making a critical analysis of the whole process with the purpose of facilitating our goal to make the human genome, as a common heritage of mankind, another legal principle of international law but without the compromise positions adopted in the case of the Law of the Sea.

---

[409]   Committee for the Study of Ethical Aspects of Human Reproduction for the International Federation of Gynecology and Obstetrics, *Patenting of Human Genes* 1997. <http://www.fi go.org/> [accessed on 20 January 2006]
[410]   Knoppers, 'Genetic Benefit Sharing', p. 49.

To begin with, there were many ideological differences between developing and developed countries and these led to significant differences in the interpretation of the legal meaning of the concept of common heritage of mankind.[411] These interpretations were never reconciled and in fact, there has never been a serious juridical consideration of the concept of common heritage of mankind to clarify them. Although a number of UN General Assembly Resolutions have tried to make the concept of common heritage of mankind a legal concept, the precise legal requirements of the concept have remained largely undefined. It was not until the 1994 Agreement that there arose near universal support for the concept.[412]

The *note verbale*[413] included as a Supplementary Item in the Agenda of the 22nd Session of the UN General Assembly by the Secretary-General in 1967 outlined the need to establish a regime to govern the deep seabed.[414] The proposal suggested both an international treaty and an international agency to regulate activities on the deep seabed.[415] The international treaty was to regulate activities on the deep seabed by establishing it as the common heritage of mankind. An international agency was to assume jurisdiction over the deep seabed, regulate and control activities undertaken on the deep seabed and enforce the treaty.

Reaction to the proposal was mixed with developing countries endorsing the principle and developed countries rejecting it. Developed countries reacted negatively to the proposal because they considered the concept too vague to have any real legal significance and because they could not imagine how the deep seabed resources could, in practical terms, belong to the world community. On the other hand, the developing countries endorsed the principle because they wanted a share in the financial benefits to be had from deep seabed mining as

---

[411] Ram Prakash Anand, *Legal Regime of the Deep Sea-Bed and the Developing Countries* (Delhi: Thompson Press, 1975), p. 205.

[412] Holmila, 'Common Heritage of Mankind in the Law of the Sea', p. 190.

[413] Arvid Pardo, Note Verbale to the Secretary-General, 22nd Sess., Annex, Mem., UN Doc. A/6695 (17 August 1967) (Request for the Inclusion of a Supplementary Item in the Agenda of the Twenty-Second Session).

[414] Arvid Pardo, 'First Statement to the First Committee of the General Assembly 1 November 1967', in *The Common Heritage of Mankind: Selected Papers on Oceans and World Order 1967–1974* (Malta: Malta University Press, 1975), pp. 39–40.

[415] Barkenbus, *Deep Seabed Resources*, pp. 32–33.

compensation for the loss of revenue which would inevitably follow after developed countries began mining the deep seabed and so buy less minerals produced by the developing countries who were the land-based producers of the seabed nodules. A second reason was related to the demand for change by developing countries embodied in the New International Economic Order[416] aimed at establishing a more equitable distribution of resources and income between developed and developing states. This goal was to be achieved by distributing the economic benefits derived from the exploitation of the deep seabed between all parties with the developed states sharing their mining technology with the developing states. As a result, the developing countries saw the concept of common heritage of mankind as a means of rectifying their economic situation.[417] Determined to push forward with the common heritage of mankind principle, the General Assembly passed Resolution 2467A with which it created the Seabed Committee,[418] which then drafted a number of resolutions, chief among them Resolution 2574D[419] and Resolution 2749.[420] The first resolution called for the creation of a moratorium on deep seabed mining until an international regime could be established. This resolution, also referred to as the Moratorium Resolution, was used by the developing countries to restrict the exploitation of the deep seabed by developed states. The resolution was particularly controversial because it ran against the *res nullius* principle espoused by many industrial

---

[416]   The NIEO was outlined at the 1964 UN Conference on Trade and Development by various declarations and was more comprehensively formulated in the '*Declaration on the Establishment of a New International Economic Order*', GA res 320 1 (SW-V1), UN GAOR, 6th Special Session, 2229th Plenary Meeting, Supplement 1, UN Doc A/9599 (1974).

[417]   Boleslaw Boczek, *Ideology and the Law of the Sea: The Challenge of the New International Economic Order*, quoted in Edward Guntrip, 'The Common Heritage of Mankind: An Adequate Regime for Managing the Deep Seabed', *Melbourne Journal of International Law*, 4:2 (2003). <http://www.mjil.law.unimelb.edu.au/issues/archive/2003(2)/02Guntrip.pdf> [accessed on 10 May 2006]

[418]   The technical name for the 'Seabed Committee' is Committee on the Peaceful Uses of the Seabed and the Ocean Floor beyond the Limits of National Jurisdiction

[419]   UNGA Res 2574 (XXIII) on the Question of the Reservation for Exclusively Peaceful Purposes of the Seabed and Ocean Floor, and the Subsoil Thereof, Underlying the High Seas Beyond the Limits of National Jurisdiction, and the Use of Their Resources in the Interests of Mankind, adopted by the General Assembly of the United Nations at its 24th Session on 15 December 1969.

[420]   UNGA Res 2749 (XXV) on the Declaration of Principles Governing the Seabed and the Ocean Floor, and the Subsoil Thereof, Beyond the Limits of National Jurisdiction, adopted by the General assembly of the United Nations at its 25th Session on 17 December 1970.

nations and, as a matter of fact, the vote on this resolution was 58 for, 29 against and 35 abstentions.[421] It was rejected by the developed, industrial nations because, it was argued, the moratorium on deep sea mining would not only hinder the future development of technologies related to deep seabed mining but also undermine the common heritage of mankind principle as no state would be able to benefit while the moratorium existed.

With the second resolution, the General Assembly adopted the Declaration of Principles in 1970. The purpose of the Declaration of Principles was to set forth the principles upon which a new and definitive legal regime could be based. The first of these principles was that the seabed and ocean floor beyond the limits of national jurisdiction were the common heritage of mankind. The second principle was that all activities regarding the exploration and exploitation of the resources of the area and other related activities were to be governed by an international regime that was to be established by an international treaty of a universal character by the UN. The regime had to provide for the equitable sharing by states in the benefits derived the exploitation of the deep seabed resources with special consideration to be given to developing countries. Unlike the Moratorium Resolution, the Declaration of Principles gained nearly universal support with 108 nations voting for, none against and 14 abstentions.[422]

Still, the Declaration of Principles did not succeed in resolving the divide between developed and developing countries, mainly because it failed to define the principle of common heritage of mankind. It was more of a compromise document, purposely uncontroversial to the point that the principles enunciated were open to wide interpretation.[423] The developed countries did not consider the Declaration to be legally binding and so it lacked any legal authority. To them it was an exercise to study the ways how the principle could, in the future, be used to govern the exploitation of the resources of the deep seabed. By contrast, the developing countries considered the Declaration as the basis of the international regime and as such made the common heritage of mankind a normative and judicially enforceable means of regulating the deep seabed.[424]

---

[421]   Barkenbus, *Deep Seabed Resources*, p. 34.

[422]   Ibid.

[423]   Edward Guntrip, 'The Common Heritage of Mankind: An Adequate Regime for Managing the Deep Seabed', *Melbourne Journal of International Law*, 4:2 (2003). <http://www.mj il.law.unimelb.edu.au/issues/archive/2003(2)/02Guntrip.pdf> [accessed on 10 April 2007]

[424]   Li, *Transfer of Technology for Deep Sea-Bed Mining*, p. 27.

With the Declaration of Principles, the General Assembly also convened the Third UN Conference on the Law of the Sea[425] in 1973 with the goal of creating a uniform codified regime to cover all aspects of the law of the sea, in particular the deep seabed.[426] It was agreed that meetings would be informal, closed to the public and with no official records. Agreement was also to be by consensus with an informal no-objection policy, often used in diplomatic negotiations, in order to avoid confrontation.[427] The UN Convention on the Law of the Sea or UNCLOS, also called the Law of the Sea Convention (LOSC) or Law of the Sea Treaty (LOST) by its critics, took place from 1973 to 1982 until finally, on 10 December 1982, the Convention was opened for signing in Montego Bay, Jamaica. Despite the controversy surrounding UNCLOS, its adoption has been hailed as one of the most significant achievements for international law. It has been referred to as a 'Constitution for the Oceans',[428] a 'world order treaty'[429] and a 'primary pillar of international law'.[430] It is unfortunate that the discussions that led to the adoption of the Declaration on the Human Genome and Human Rights by the UNESCO General Conference on 11 November 1997 did not generate the same interest among the delegates as did Pardo's proposal on the deep seabed.

To start with, the question of the resources of the deep seabed was a matter of concern for both developed and developing states—in fact it was the developing states that had more to lose if the resources of the deep seabed and ocean floor were not made the common heritage of mankind. The situation is very different with the human genome when many of the developing states are not

---

[425]   The Third United Nations Conference on the Law of the Sea held its first session in 1973 and worked for several months each year until it finally adopted the United Nations Convention on the Law of the Sea in 1982.

[426]   Ibid., 37.

[427]   Susan Peterson, 'The Common Heritage of Mankind?', *Environment*, 22:1 (1980), pp. 6–11.

[428]   Tommy T.B. Koh, 'A Constitution of the Oceans', in *United Nations Convention on the Law of the Sea 1982: A Commentary*, ed. by Myron H. Nordquist (Dordrecht: Martinus Nijhoff Publishers, 1985), pp. 11–16.

[429]   Christian Tomuschat, *Obligations Arising for States Without or Against Their Will*, quoted in Peter S. Prows, *Tough Love: The Dramatic Birth and Looming Demise of UNCLOS Property Law*, New York University Public Law and Legal Theory Working Papers, Paper 30 (2006), p. 1. < http://ssrn.com/abstract=918458> [accessed 15 June 2008]

[430]   David J. Bederman, *Counterintuiting Countermeasures*, quoted in Peter S. Prows, *Tough Love: The Dramatic Birth and Looming Demise of UNCLOS Property Law*, New York University Public Law and Legal Theory Working Papers, Paper 30 (2006), p. 1. < http://ssrn.com/abst ract=918458> [accessed 15 June 2008]

really in any way directly involved in the genomic research that is centred on the human genome—suffice to say that more than 4000 genes, or 20% of the almost 24,000 human genes, have been claimed by US patents! At the same time, the developed states never really took the Declaration seriously—partly because of the terminology used that referred to the human genome as the 'heritage of humanity, in a symbolic form'. As already explained, this terminology was used so as to avoid a reductionist approach to the human genome that did not consider the metaphysical implications of the genome. But unfortunately this terminology introduced an element of ambiguity surrounding the intention behind the Declaration in deciding to refrain from stating, categorically, that the human genome was the common heritage of humanity.

The most controversial part of UNCLOS[431] was Part XI with many of the developed states declaring, before the conclusion of the Conference, that they were not happy with the provisions related to seabed mining. Referring to the seabed as the 'Area' which is defined as 'the seabed, ocean floor and subsoil thereof, beyond the limits of national jurisdiction',[432] the Conference declared the 'Area' as being governed by the common heritage of mankind with the prohibition imposed on all states to claim or exercise 'sovereignty or sovereign rights' and natural or juridical persons 'appropriating any part thereof'.[433] Article 140 (1) provided that all activities must be undertaken for the benefit of mankind as a whole with special consideration to be given to the interests and needs of developing countries. That the use of the 'Area' was to be exclusively for peaceful purposes was provided for in Article 141, while Article 137 (2) gave the International Seabed Authority jurisdiction to act on behalf of mankind as a whole in whom the resources of the 'Area' were vested.

Among the countries that were not satisfied with the provisions of Part XI and refused to sign UNCLOS was the US, claiming as its main reservation to the Convention that it would deter the future development of deep seabed mining for mineral resources.[434] But the biggest problem for the US was the International Seabed Authority which did not give the Americans an adequate role in the decision-making processes and had the faculty to allow amendments without the US's prior approval. Other US objections were to the mandatory transfer of

---

[431] United Nations Convention on the Law of the Sea (UNCLOS), Montego Bay, 10 December 1982.
[432] UNCLOS, 1982, Article 1 (1).
[433] Ibid., Article 137 (1).

technology provided for by the Convention, the questionability of the way mining contracts would be granted and the artificial limitations that could be imposed on seabed production which could exert some financial burdens on the
US economy.[435]

It did not come to a surprise to most of the delegates that the US refused to
sign UNCLOS since it had most to lose. The US was not ready to relinquish its
dominant role in matters that concerned the seabed, ocean floor and subsoil beyond national jurisdiction. For the same reason it refused to accept the International Seabed Authority because in doing so, it would have to accept to be one
player among many! The question is whether the US will react the same way if,
like the seabed, ocean floor and subsoil beyond national jurisdiction, the human
genome is made the common heritage of mankind with the provisions of UN-
CLOS Part XI, which would entail, among other things, relinquishing its dominant role in the patenting of the human genome which at the present amounts to
around 20% of the total number of human genes? The second question is
whether the US will be ready to delegate its dominant role as a policy-maker in
the biotechnology industry to an authority established on the same lines as the
International Seabed Authority but with jurisdiction over the human genome?
And the third question concerns the readiness of the US to give special consideration to the interests and needs of the developing countries in the use of biotechnology for research on the human genome?

These are the primary concerns that must pre-empt any serious endeavour,
on an international political level, to make the human genome a legal principle
of international law. Take the situation faced by Brazil when because it refused
to allow product patents for pharmaceuticals, the US government, on the insti-
gation of Pharmaceutical Manufacturers of America, imposed a $39 million tar-
iff on imports of Brazilian pharmaceuticals! Brazil does not allow patents on
pharmaceuticals because it is common practice among pharmaceutical companies not to manufacture a new product for a tropical disease because of the absence of a profitable market. So Brazil's solution to this situation was to allow
process patents but not on pharmaceutical products.[436]

[435]   Guntrip, 'The Common Heritage of Mankind', p. 9.
[436]   Sigrid Sterckx, 'Lack of Access to Essential Drugs: A Story of Continuing Global Failure, with
        Particular Attention to the Role of Patents', in *Ethics and Law of Intellectual Property: Current
        Problems in Politics, Science and Technology*, ed. by Christian Lenk, Nils Hoppe and Roberto
        Andorno (Aldershot: Ashgate, 2007), pp. 175–97.

As expected, many developed countries did not sign UNCLOS, jeopardizing in the process, the efforts of many countries to formulate a codified Law of the Sea on the basis of the common heritage of mankind principle. Several developed countries, including the US, France, Italy, Japan, the Soviet Union, the UK and West Germany, passed national legislation to provide for the licensing of exploration and exploitation on the deep seabed outside the UNCLOS regime.[437] A Reciprocating States Regime was also established in order to avoid the overlapping of licenses issued by the different legislating states.[438]

The problem is that the establishment of this regime by the countries that opposed UNCLOS does not augur well for our project of making the human genome the common heritage of mankind. A similar arrangement might be made between countries that are opposed to relinquishing the exclusive proprietary rights awarded to them by the patenting system as presently operated even though, to the detriment of the interests of all mankind, the system is conducive to maintaining the *tragedy of the anti-commons*, as already explained.

In order to put an end to this impasse, the UN General Assembly set about modifying the provisions of UNCLOS to which the developed nations had the greatest opposition which included the transfer of technology, the training of personnel and the decision-making process of the International Seabed Authority. Consequently the UN General Assembly drafted the 1994 Implementation Agreement that was to be interpreted as a single instrument with Part XI of the UNCLOS Convention. In the case of any inconsistencies between the 1994 Agreement and Part XI, the 1994 Agreement was to prevail. Any subsequent ratifications of UNCLOS bound a state to the 1994 Agreement while states could not accede to the 1994 Agreement without also adopting UNCLOS.[439]

The 1994 Agreement achieved almost universal consensus but at the cost of sacrificing most of the essential elements of the concept of common heritage of mankind as proposed by Arvid Pardo and as articulated in the original Maltese

---

[437]   Deep Seabed Hard Minerals Resources Act 1980 (USA), Law on the Exploration and Exploitation of the Mineral Resources of the Deep Seabed 1985 (Italy), Law on Interim Measures for Deep Seabed Mining 1983 (Japan), Edict on Provisional Measures to Regulate Soviet Enterprises for the Exploration and Exploitation of Mineral Resources 1982 (USSR), Deep Sea Mining (Temporary Provisions) Act 1981 (UK), Act of Interim Regulation of Deep Seabed Mining 1982 (Federal republic of Germany).

[438]   R.R. Churchill and A.V. Lowe, *The Law of the Sea* (Manchester: Manchester University Press, 1999), pp. 232–35.

[439]   Guntrip, 'The Common Heritage of Mankind', p. 10.

Draft.[440] So, even though today one might argue that the common heritage of mankind binds a majority of states through UNCLOS, it is only the issue of regime management that has achieved sufficient clarification to attain legal force. One of the substantive elements of the common heritage of mankind that was brushed aside was Pardo's idea that all natural resources, living or non-living, existing beyond the 200-mile limit would be managed by international institutions so as to ensure the equitable sharing by all states of the benefits derived from the development of these resources and in order to take into particular consideration the interests and needs of poor countries. The same fate was met by the proviso, in the original draft proposal, that the coastal state, within the 200-mile limit, would be obliged to make contributions for the financial benefits derived from the extension of its rights on the resources contained therein.[441] The almost universal consensus was bought at the cost of introducing a 200-mile 'Exclusive Economic Zone' that permitted countries to exercise sovereign rights over resources within this area—this means that the Treaty actually increased the sovereignty rights of countries! So it is fair to say that while the concept of common heritage of mankind, as originally envisaged by Arvid Pardo and with the backing of the developing countries of the G-77, symbolized the interests, needs, hopes and aspirations of a large number of poor people who were ready to strive hard for a New International Economic Order, it ended by representing the interests of an increasingly dominating free market economy that was the anti-thesis of the concept:

> While NIEO aspirations and the common heritage remain linked philosophically, the prospects for realizing either have dimmed markedly over the past three decades. It is true that the CHMP has emerged as a legitimate treaty-based principle of international law. That the UN Law of the Sea Convention entered into force in 1994 attests to as much. Even so, the CHMP still lacks acceptance as a customary legal norm sustained and substantiated by state practice.[442]

Although it is fair to say that the concept of the common heritage of mankind has normative value under international treaty law in the terms provided by the

---

[440]   Pardo, *The Common Heritage of Mankind*, p. 381.

[441]   Tullio Scovazzi, The Concept of Common Heritage of Mankind and the Resources of the Seabed Beyond the Limits of National Jurisdiction, p. 5. <http://www.iadb.org/.../Seminario_AU SPINTAL_2006_04_Scovazzi.pdf> [accessed on April 20 2007]

[442]   Christopher Joynor, *International Law in the 21st Century: Rules for Global Governance* (Lanham, MD: Rowman and Littlefield, 2005), p. 244.

Law of the Sea Convention, it has failed to attain normative value under customary international law because with the developed nations' opposition to UN-CLOS III and the subsequent compromise position of the 1994 Agreement adopted by the UN to get them on board, the concept was denied a free-standing, self-evident definition. As things now stand, its meaning is determined by the way it has been implemented in the deep seabed area in the Law of the Sea Convention. And, despite its flaws, the Law of the Sea remains the blueprint for making the human genome, as common heritage of mankind, a legal principle of international law. That the concept of common heritage of mankind has attained normative value under international treaty law is a success in itself but the end result is not what Pardo had intended—it is a travesty of the Pardosian concept. Most opposition came from the US that is considered to be one of the world leaders in ocean policy and which, to this day, has not ratified the Treaty![443]

2.8 The International Management of the Human Genome as a Common Heritage of Mankind

The next section of our study will be focused on the international management of the human genome as a common heritage of mankind. Different proposals were put forward by the developing and developed countries when they were discussing how, in practical terms, the resources of the deep seabed could be managed by an international agency. All of these proposals can offer us some insight on how we can create the best possible international management structure for the human genome as a common heritage of mankind. We will start by examining the proposals put forward by the developing and developed countries for an International Seabed Authority together with the reasons behind these proposals. We will then discuss the relevance of these proposals to the main object of our concern which is the human genome. In the end we will make our own proposal for the international management of the human genome as a common heritage of mankind.

The lengthy negotiations that followed Pardo's proposal to make the resources of the deep seabed the common heritage of mankind eventually led to

---

[443] On May 15, President George W. Bush publicly urged the US Senate to support the Treaty and to vote in favour of ratification.

the establishment of the International Seabed Authority whose creation was provided by Section 4 of Part XI of UNCLOS.[444] Initially, the developing countries intended this International Seabed Authority to be an international seabed mining entity with the exclusive responsibility for the management of the resources of the deep seabed. All other mining companies, both private and public, were to be barred from carrying out any form of mining activity in waters that were beyond the limits of national jurisdiction.

A similar international authority could be established for the human genome which, initially, would be entrusted with reforming the patent system in the interests of the common good.[445] As explained earlier in our study, the human genome stands both for the full set of genes of each individual and for the entire range of genes that constitute the human species. In making the human genome the common heritage of mankind, five fundamental principles of the concept must be taken into consideration, namely,

i.   The human genome must not be subject to appropriation of any kind whether public or private;

ii.   The management of the human genome must be carried out by and on behalf of all humanity or by 'trustee' representatives;

iii. Any benefits flowing from such management must be shared amongst all humanity;

iv.   The use of the human genome must be limited to peaceful purposes and,

v.   Scientific research on the human genome must be carried out freely so long as the human genome is not compromised in any way and the results are openly published for the benefit of all humanity.

These prerequisites for making the human genome the common heritage of mankind are in sharp contrast with the patent system that, as Seth Shulman has explained, is setting the stage for 'a long term intellectual property disaster' considering the wide range of property rights associated with the patenting of DNA and human genes that the system supports. Shulman proposes five steps in order to prevent this disaster, namely (i) to create an intellectual property sanctuary where intellectual property would not apply; (ii) to declare a moratorium on further gene patenting; (iii) to institute a compulsory licensing system so as to make sure that the patentee would not be able to exclude others from having access to

---

[444]   UNCLOS 1982, Article 156 (1).
[445]   Lebacqz, 'Who "Owns" Cells and Tissues?', pp. 356–68 (p. 363).

knowledge related to the patent; (iv) to set up a committee that will establish policy around gene patents and, (v) to put concerns about public health and the equitable sharing of health-related products before commercial gain.[446] These proposals could be implemented by an International Human Genome Authority established under the auspices of the UN with the dual mandate of (i) making the concept of common heritage of mankind as applied to the human genome a legal principle of international law, and (ii) overhauling the patent system by putting community interests before individual interests.

Returning to the negotiations that led to the establishment of the International Seabed Authority, the developed countries were in total disagreement with the proposed model of the developing countries that assigned exclusive responsibility for the exploitation of the seabed resources in the waters beyond national jurisdiction to the International Seabed Authority. They would have preferred the International Seabed Authority to be an International Registry of mining activities in the waters beyond national jurisdiction without any of the executive powers that the developing countries wanted to assign to the Authority so as to be able to regulate the exploitation of the seabed by private and public mining companies.[447]

The idea of an International Registry for mining activities in the waters beyond national jurisdiction is more in line with considering the resources of the deep seabed and ocean floor as a *common concern of mankind* rather than as a common heritage of mankind.[448] As already explained in our study, the fundamental difference between the two concepts is the issue of non-appropriation that is applicable to a common heritage but not to a *common concern of mankind*.

Still, the idea of an International Registry can be borrowed from the Law of the Sea negotiations and be made applicable to the human genome as an International Registry for human genomic research that would eventually replace the patent system. Under the auspices of the UN, an International Human Genome Registry could be established with the purpose of making all the uses of genomic information registered with its international genetic databank freely available to both private and public companies that show interest in this infor-

---

[446]   Ibid.
[447]   Churchill and Lowe, *Law of the Sea*, pp. 228–29.
[448]   UNGA Res. 43/53 on the Protection of Global Climate for Present and Future Generations of Mankind, adopted on 6 December 1988.

mation subject to a reasonable fee. Part of the fee can be transferred to the researcher[449] while the rest of the fee will be utilized in the interests of all mankind. In this way, the special rights awarded to researchers will be reconciled with the interests of all mankind in the spirit of the concept of common heritage of mankind.

When the International Seabed Authority was established with UNCLOS, a compromise position was found as a way of bridging the gap between the developed countries who wanted the International Seabed Authority to run things on the basis of a free-market system and the developing countries who wanted a more stable management in terms of economic and environmental affairs with special consideration given to their interests and needs. This political compromise was reached with the method of operation of the 'Enterprise' that functions as the business arm of the International Seabed Authority with responsibility for mining activities by the Authority.[450] The Enterprise was not to have exclusive responsibility for all mining activities in the waters beyond national jurisdiction as had been originally proposed by the developing countries. On the contrary, a 'parallel system'[451] was adopted whereby states and private companies would be able to carry out mining activities alongside the Enterprise as long as they were respectful of the rules, regulations and procedures of the Authority.[452] This way the responsibility for mining activities was shared with both states and private companies. The Enterprise was not the legislative arm of the International Seabed Authority. This was the responsibility of the 'Assembly'[453] that was to determine general policies while responsibility for decisions on which specific policies and activities were to be pursued by the Authority rested with the 'Council'.[454]

The same management structure of the International Seabed Authority can be applied to the human genome as a common heritage of mankind. First, an International Human Genome Authority could be set up, comparable to the International Seabed Authority. The responsibility of this International Human Genome Authority would be to manage the human genome as a common heritage of all mankind. All States Parties would form part of the Assembly in a

---

[449]   Ryuichi, 'Human Genome as Common Heritage of Mankind', pp. 59–63.

[450]   UNCLOS 1982, Article 170.

[451]   The operational details of the 'Parallel System' are to be found in UNCLOS 1982, Annexes III and IV.

[452]   UNCLOS 1982, Article 153.

[453]   UNCLOS 1982, Articles 156(2), 159; 1994 IA, Annex, Section 1, para. 12.

[454]   UNCLOS 1982, Article 162.

similar way to the constituted Assembly of the International Seabed Authority. However, in the case of the International Human Genome Authority, the representation would not be of one member for each state as in the case of the International Seabed Authority, but rather a method of proportional representation should be adopted. The reason for this is that as the International Human Genome Authority will be responsible for managing the human genome on behalf of all mankind it would be fair to have proportionate representation for all the people who are comprised by the States Parties—in other words, it does not make sense for the people of Malta and the people of the US to have equal representation. There would also be the Council of the International Human Genome Authority composed of members nominated by all States Parties and elected to the Council by the Assembly.

In the course of our research we have come to believe that in issues related to the human genome, politicians should not be the people making decisions on behalf and in the interests of all mankind. The fact that their parliamentary responsibilities are directly related to their level of popularity with the general electorate constitutes a direct conflict of interest when they may choose political opportunism over political altruism in the interests of all mankind. For these reasons, politicians should not be allowed to be part of the Council. Members of the Council should be elected by the Assembly after being nominated by their respective governments. The members chosen to sit on the Council should be learned individuals who can guide the Assembly in managing the human genome as the common heritage of mankind. Accordingly their expertise should cover the whole spectrum of knowledge that is indispensable to perform such a task. The Council should also be able to consult 'Committees of Experts' appositely appointed by the Assembly to advice the Council when necessary.

The International Human Genome Authority, unlike the International Seabed Authority, would have more than one operational arm which can be referred to as 'Genome-Enterprises'. The European Patent Office, under the auspices of the International Human Genome Authority, could become 'Genome-Enterprise (Europe)' with responsibility for the member states of the European Union. The United States Patent and Trademark Office, again under the auspices of the International Human Genome Authority, could become 'Genome-Enterprise (US)'. The role of the Genome-Enterprises would be to carry out Research and Development (R&D) under the auspices of the International Human Genome Authority. The establishment of the Genome-Enterprises would not mean that private and public sector R&D companies would have to stop operations. They would still be able to perform R&D but only as subcontractors for the Genome-Enterprise to which they would be affiliated, as long as they respected the rules, terms and conditions established by the International Human Genome Authority. So with the human genome, private and public companies that chose to carry our R&D would not be allowed to do so independently of the Enterprise as provided for by the International Seabed Authority, but rather under the direct management of the Genome-Enterprises of the International Human Genome Authority. This arrangement is more consonant with the idea of international management that was first proposed by the developing countries. In fact the original idea of constituting the Enterprise came from three Latin American delegates, Sergio Thompson Flores of Brazil,[455] Alvaro de Soto of Peru[456] and Lennox Ballah of Trinidad and Tobago.[457] So in effect with the human genome, the compromise position adopted to accommodate the developed countries would not be sustained.

Those companies that chose to invest heavily in this kind of R&D would be compensated accordingly by established rules to be determined by the Assembly. These private and public subcontractors will be obliged to keep the Genome-Enterprises informed of any new biomedical inventions and the biotechnology used to arrive at such inventions. If the Genome-Enterprises are unable to acquire the biotechnology being used by subcontractors on the open market than the subcontractors would be obliged to transfer that biotechnology to the Genome-Enterprises on fair and reasonable commercial terms and conditions. If the subcontractors are unable to transfer the biotechnology because they are not the owners, then they must provide written assurance that the biotechnology will be transferred to the Genome-Enterprises by the owners on fair and reasonable commercial terms and conditions. If no such transfer is made, then the subcontractors would be barred from using that biotechnology and from claiming any financial benefit from the biomedical inventions made using that particular biotechnology.

With the establishment of the International Human Genome Authority, the Assembly, Council and Genome-Enterprises, the five essential elements of the concept of common heritage of mankind can be effectively applied to the human genome. First of all, the human genome and all biomedical inventions would

---

[455]   John J. Logue (ed.), *The Fate of the Oceans* (Pennsylvania: Villanova University Press, 1972), pp. 195–200.

[456]   Ibid., pp. 113–20.

[457]   Ibid., pp. 188–92.

become the common heritage of mankind and therefore no longer subject to appropriation by any private or public entity as is happening at the moment with the way the patent system is being run. Secondly, the human genome and all biomedical inventions would be managed for the benefit of all mankind. Third, the International Human Genome Authority will be able to ensure that the developing countries will share in the benefits to be derived from the management of the human genome the same as the developed countries. Fourth, the human genome and biomedical inventions will only be used for exclusively peaceful purposes. And finally, scientific research on the human genome will be freely carried out and the results of this research freely disseminated for the benefit of all humanity.

2.9   Extrapolating with the Common Heritage of Mankind

The lessons learnt from the UNCLOS-prototype can be used to launch the International Human Genome Authority without the plethora of difficulties experienced in the difficult birth of UNCLOS III that was only eventually made possible with the anomalous 1994 Agreement. Several commentators have proposed ways how the concept of common heritage of mankind could be applied to the human genome. A common thread among these contributors is the idea that the human genome is a common natural resource that must be developed and protected for the benefit of all humanity. Insights from environmental ethics have been applied to the debate on the human genome as common heritage of mankind with particular concern being focussed on the question of whether the genome should be made patentable subject matter and if so, in what way and to what extent.

But first there are lessons to be learnt from attempts already made by the international community to claim, as the common heritage of mankind, outer space, the moon and Antarctica. The discussions that led to the Outer space Treaty of 1967,[458] the Moon Agreement of 1979[459] and the Antarctic Treaty of 1959[460] are particularly relevant to the human genome debate on the issue of

---

[458]   Treaty on Principles Governing the Activities of States in the Exploration and Use of Outer Space, Including the Moon and Other Celestial Bodies, adopted by the General Assembly of the United Nations at its 21st Session on 19 December 1966. UNGA Res. 2222 (XXI).

[459]   Agreement Governing the Activities of States on the Moon and Other Celestial Bodies, adopted by the General Assembly of the United Nations at its 34th Session on 14 December 1979. UNGA Res. 34/68.

[460]   Antarctic Treaty (1959). Antarctic Connection. <http://www.antarcticconnection.com/antarcti c/treaty/index.shtml> [accessed on 20 January 2006]

common heritage versus patentability. As in the case of the Law of the Seabed Convention, the concept of the common heritage of mankind as incorporated in these international documents is a parody of the Pardosian concept of common heritage that should comprise the four fundamental principles of (i) non-appropriation, (ii) management by and on behalf of all humanity, (iii) sharing of benefits amongst all humanity and, (iv) exclusive use for peaceful purposes. Of the three international documents, it is only the Moon Agreement that specifically mentions the concept of common heritage of mankind in the same terms as the Law of the Sea Convention of 1982.[461] The Outer Space Treaty does not go so far but stops at proclaiming that, as the moon and other celestial bodies are the 'province of all mankind', they should not be appropriated and all exploration and exploitation must be carried out for the benefit of all countries and for peaceful purposes.[462] Furthermore, while the Outer Space Treaty does not contain any provision for the establishment of an international regime, the Moon Agreement provides both for the establishment of such an international regime and for the appropriate procedures that may be necessary to carry out the exploitation of the natural resources of the moon when such exploitation becomes materially and financially feasible.[463] Finally, the Outer Space Treaty[464] and the Moon Agreement[465] exclude the possibility of appropriation, by claims of sovereignty of 'outer space', the 'moon' and' celestial bodies'.

It must be noted that although the Moon Agreement, after a first reading, may appear to endorse a concept of the common heritage of mankind similar to that found in the Law of the Sea Convention of 1982, it actually confines itself to applying the concept of common heritage of mankind to the States Parties to the Agreement[466] as regards both the establishment of an international regime and equitable sharing of resources:

> An equitable sharing by all States Parties in the benefits derived from those resources, whereby the interests and needs of the developing countries, as well as the efforts of those

---

[461]   Moon Agreement, Articles 1 and 11.
[462]   Outer Space Treaty, Articles 1, 2, 4.
[463]   Moon Agreement Article 11(5).
[464]   Outer Space Treaty Article 2.
[465]   Moon Agreement Article 11(2).
[466]   Ibid., Article 11 (5).

countries which have contributed either directly or indirectly to the exploration of the moon, shall be given special consideration.[467]

This makes the international management and exploitation of the moon and its resources an exclusive and potentially secretive affair that does not tally with the concerns expressed by the majority of the developing countries in the context of the New International Economic Order. The same can be said of the Antarctic Treaty[468] that was signed by 12 states on 1 December 1959 and a further 14 states with the last state to sign the Treaty being Estonia on 17 May 2001.[469] The primary goal of the Treaty has been to ensure, in the interests of all mankind, that Antarctica will continue to be used for only peaceful purposes and that it will never become the 'scene or object of international discord'.[470] Accordingly, the Treaty prohibits any form of military activity unless it is for scientific purposes,[471] and any nuclear explosions together with the disposal of radioactive waste material.[472] In the spirit of the concept of common heritage of mankind, the Treaty promotes scientific research and any exchange of data[473] and, paradoxically, holds all territorial claims in abeyance.[474] Technically, the Antarctic is not the common heritage of mankind because it is 'owned' by 44 Antarctic

---

[467] Ibid., Article 11 (7) (d).

[468] Antarctic Treaty (1959). Antarctic Connection. <http://www.antarcticconnection.com/antarcti c/treaty/index.shtml> [accessed on 20 January 2006]

[469] The first States to sign the Treaty, referred to as 'Parties to the Treaty' were twelve nations that were active in the Antarctic during the International Geophysical Year of 1957–58. This original group of twelve States was joined by fifteen additional States that, like the original twelve Parties to the Treaty, became Consultative States by acceding to the Treaty and by conducting substantial scientific activity in Antarctica. Another eighteen States have since acceded to the Treaty by agreeing to abide by the Treaty and may attend the consultative meetings as observers. The Treaty has been augmented by Recommendations adopted at Consultative Meetings, by the Protocol on environmental Protection to the Antarctic Treaty (Madrid 1991) and by two separate conventions dealing with the Conservation of Antarctic Seals (London 1972) and the Conservation of Antarctic Marine Living Resources (Canberra 1980). The Antarctic treaty Consultative Meeting is held annually during which a meeting of the Committee of Environmental Protection is also held. At both meeting the Scientific Committee on Antarctic research is an observer and provides scientific advice as requested by the participants at the meetings.

[470] Preamble to Antarctic treaty (1959).

[471] Antarctic Treaty Article 1.

[472] Ibid., Article 5.

[473] Ibid., Article 3.

[474] Ibid., Article 4.

Treaty nations that roughly represent only two-thirds of the world's human population. As things stand, the concept of common heritage of mankind has no
credence in Antarctica.[475] However, it can become the common heritage of mankind if a truly international regime is established with the purpose of exploiting
its resources for the benefit of all mankind. Malaysia and Antigua and Barbuda
are two nations, not parties to the Antarctic Treaty, that are successfully engaging the UN General Assembly to set in motion the process to make Antarctica,
the only continent with no nations, a veritable common heritage of mankind![476]
    It is significant to our debate on the issue of the human genome and the
common heritage of mankind that as of 1 January 2008, while 98 states ratified
the Outer Space Treaty, only 11 states chose to ratify the Moon Agreement. Developed states had no problem signing the Outer space Treaty because, in their
view, it was consonant with their views on free markets but the same could not
be said of the Moon Agreement that unlike Part XI of the Law of the Sea Convention of 1982 which is part of a package deal together with the 1994 Agreement stands by itself. The difficulty stems from the developed countries' reluctance to enframe the concept of common heritage of mankind, in all of its essential elements, in international law which is binding for all states. The Antarctic
question is symptomatic of this *laissez faire* attitude in many of the developed
countries' thinking that is an obstacle to implementing a New International Economic Order that will give developing countries a greater say in world affairs
with a view to generating a more equitable distribution of natural resources
among all mankind comprising also future generations. It is disturbing to think
that while many developed countries found no difficulty in signing the Outer
Space Treaty because it does not deny the free market philosophy, the Moon
Agreement has been put on the back burner and the Antarctic Treaty remains an
agreement of convenience among forty-four nations to refrain from exploiting
the region presumably until it becomes more convenient to do so!
    A parallel situation is to be found in the area of biotechnology when phar-
maceutical companies and other organizations from both the private and public
sector are reluctant to consider the human genome as the common heritage of
mankind because of the financial setbacks that may result from the regulation of

475   P.J. Beck, 'The United Nations and Antarctica, 2005: The End of the 'Question of Antarctica?',
        Polar Record, 42:3 (2006), 217–27.
476   Gillian D. Triggs (ed), *The Antarctic Treaty Regime* (Cambridge: Cambridge University Press,
        1987), pp. 53–54.

gene DNA patenting by an international regime such as the proposed International Human Genome Authority. The governance of the human genome should be regulated by a Human Genome Agreement that, like the Moon Agreement, will stand by itself and like the Outer Space Treaty be ratified by the majority of states, both developed and developing ones.

Several commentators have in recent years proposed different ways how the human genome could be considered the common heritage of mankind. Their contributions are able to shed light from various angles on the human genome's suitability as a common heritage of mankind and in this respect provide food for thought in the as yet uncharted course towards establishing an international regime for protecting and developing the human genome on behalf of all mankind.

2.10 Further Reaches of the Genome

For Professor Ossorio, the oceans were regarded as *res nullius* until they were declared the common heritage of mankind by the Law of the Sea Convention.[477] Like the moon and Antarctica, she believes that the human genome should be made an essential component of the common heritage of mankind and she lists a number of reasons to justify her proposal. These reasons are centred on the intergenerational and intragenerational continuum of genes between generations and between individuals and their ancestors, descendants and siblings. Genes represent a connection between all members of the human species while the human genome is the embodiment of human evolution, constituting a bridge between the past, present and the future. To this effect, Professor Ossorio remarks that, '...people who do not hold genetic reductionist or determinist views may feel that something deeply important is reflected or embodied in our genomes'.[478]

In her article, *The Human Genome: Common Sense or Legal Nonsense*, Ossorio contributes to the debate on the human genome as a component of the common heritage of mankind by proposing a modern version of the stewardship model in the form of a 'Public Trust Doctrine' that is an extension of the *res publicae* category of public property in the Roman Law tradition. There are a number of conceptual underpinnings that justify holding the human genome as a public trust. First of all, human genomic knowledge is of intrinsic importance

---

[477]　Pilar N. Ossorio, 'Common Heritage Arguments and the Patenting of DNA', in *Perspectives on Gene Patenting: Religion, Science and Industry in Dialogue*, ed. by A.R. Chapman (Washington D.C.: American Association for the Advancement of Science, 1988), pp. 89–110.

[478]　Ossorio, 'The Human Genome as Common Heritage', pp. 425–39 (p. 425).

to all of mankind and so it stands to reason that everyone wants the liberty to be able to make use of this knowledge. Secondly, as the biomedical inventions and other benefits that are derived from the study of the human genome are the direct result of the study of nature, they must be made available to all those who show an interest in them. Finally, the public was kept informed of the progress being achieved in the various HGPs as it was agreed from the start, by the major policy makers, that in evaluating policy decisions concerning human DNA, there should be 'broad public input with a robust deliberative process'.[479]

The Common Heritage Duties Doctrine is the new jacket that Professor Ossorio puts on the human genome with a nod in the direction of the fair distribution of duties and burdens rather than the fair distribution of benefits. Immanent in this doctrine is the value of stewardship that assigns human beings fiduciary duties towards other human beings and the non-human natural world.[480] As applied to the human genome, these duties may entail adopting a normative stance to refrain from adopting a reductionist approach to the human genome so as to preserve and protect it for future generations. As Ossorio comments in her article, members of the Council of Europe have argued that '...human rights to life and dignity entail the right to inherit a genome that has not been artificially altered'.[481] The importance of such a policy statement cannot be underestimated considering the dual nature of the human genome. First, while each human genome stands for a unique individual, the genome was formed from other genomes and will help form other genomes because each of us shares parts of our genomes with parents, siblings and family. So, the information contained within an individual genome has both a private and public nature because it is relevant not only to the person who stands for the particular genome but also for all other genomes that helped form the genome and that may be formed from the genome in question.

The Common Heritage Duties Doctrine is an extension of the Public Trust Doctrine that is considered to be a cornerstone of modern environmental law. The Public Trust Doctrine mainly relates to issues of ownership and protection

---

[479] Ibid., p. 427.

[480] Kemal Baslar, *The Concept of Common Heritage of Mankind in International Law*, quoted in Ossorio, 'The Human Genome as Common Heritage', pp. 425–39 (p. 431).

[481] Parliamentary Assembly of the Council of Europe Recommendation 934 (1982) on Genetic Engineering.

and/or use of essential natural and cultural resources. Its basic tenet is that certain essential resources, because of their unique characteristics, should be held in trust on behalf of all citizens. A government authority, appointed as a trustee, assumes the fiduciary duty of stewardship of the essential resources in question for the benefit of all mankind.[482] The Common Heritage Duties Doctrine was first codified in the Convention for the Protection of Cultural Property in the Event of Armed Conflict[483] and in the Convention for the Protection of the World Cultural and Natural Heritage.[484] The basic rationale underpinning these two Conventions was that if the 'greatness and goodness of a people'[485] could be encapsulated in a product of man's creative ingenuity, then 'awe-inspiring artefacts are important for fostering creative efforts among members of present and future generations',[486] and must therefore be protected and preserved by the present generation for posterity.

David R. Resnik, like Pilar Ossorio, chooses not to think of the human genome as the common heritage of mankind but rather as a common resource.[487] Taking the cue from environmental ethics, he points out that from such a consideration of the human genome, the duties of stewardship and justice must be met by the present generation on behalf of both current and future generations.[488] The main duties of stewardship to the human genome comprise its protection from harm and its development for the benefit of all mankind. Among the serious threats that, according to Resnik, pose a real danger to the human genome are the loss of genetic diversity and the adverse effects that can be produced as a result of man-induced genetic mutations. More specifically, the duties of stewardship entail avoiding eugenic implications such as forced sterilization, restricted procreation, ethnic cleansing, genocide, genetic discrimination and other

---

[482]   Patricia Kameri-Mbote, 'The Use of the Public Trust Doctrine in Environmental Law', *Law, Environment and Development Journal*, 3/2 (2007), 197–201 (p. 195) <http://www.lead-journal.org/content/07195.pdf> [accessed 5 July 2008]

[483]   Convention for the Protection of Cultural Property in the Event of Armed Conflict, adopted at The Hague (Netherlands) on 14 May 1954.

[484]   Convention Concerning the Protection of the World Cultural and Natural Heritage, adopted by the General Conference of UNESCO at its 17th Session on 16 November 1972.

[485]   Ossorio, 'The Human Genome as Common Heritage', pp. 430–31.

[486]   Ibid., p. 431.

[487]   David R. Resnik, 'The Human Genome: Common Resource but not Common Heritage', in *Ethics for Life Scientists*, ed. by Michiel Korthals and Robert J. Borges (Dordrecht: Springer, 2004), pp. 197–210.

[488]   Resnik, *Owning the Genome*, p. 82.

immoral activities that may be pursued under the pretence of purifying the human genome. Cloning, germ-line manipulation and other similar activities which are considered morally unacceptable by the majority of people should also be banned as they posed a significant risk to the human genome proper and to future generations.[489]

Duties of justice to a common resource demand that it is used justly and fairly. As applied to the human genome, duties of justice would entail, among other things, taking precautionary measures to prevent or minimize the potential negative effects of patents on discovery and innovation.[490] At one end of the spectrum is the ban on some types of patents such as patents in DNA. At the other end of the spectrum, there is the implementation of policies that could minimize the threats posed by biotechnology patents. Resnik suggests several ways how to deal with such threats such as raising the bar on the various conditions which must be met for awarding a patent or restricting the scope of patents, even though these preventive measures provide no certain guarantee that new inventions will not face 'patent thickets' or exhortative license fees.

Resnik and others have suggested that the anti-commons effect of the patenting system could be overcome by creating a 'biotechnology patent pool' or 'patent clearinghouse' which, together with cross-licensing, could effectively become one-stop-shops offering non-exclusive licenses to research institutes involved in the biotechnology sector.[491] As a patent holder has the negative right to exclude others from making, using or commercializing his invention, non-exclusive licensing will ensure that vital genomic knowledge will remain in the public domain for the benefit of all mankind.[492] The patent pool should be designed in such a manner that while transaction costs are kept to a minimum, the pool itself will be able to negotiate licenses on behalf of its members and thus spare the licensees from having to negotiate with several patent holders. As the public and private sectors already hold patents on materials and methods in biotechnology, Resnik proposes that the patent pool should be an independent, non-profit body comprising private corporations and private universities as well as public universities and government agencies modelled on already existing copyright agencies such as the Copyright Clearinghouse Centre.[493]

---

[489]   Resnik, 'The Human Genome: Common Resource but not Common Heritage', pp. 197–210.

[490]   Resnik, 'A Biotechnology Patent Pool'.

[491]   Thumm, 'Patents for Genetic Inventions', 1410–17.

[492]   David R. Resnik, 'DNA Patents and Human Dignity', *Journal of Law, Medicine and Ethics*, 29:2 (2001), pp. 152–65.

[493]   Resnik, 'A Biotechnology Patent Pool'.

2.11 Launching the Global Governance of the Human Genome

The mandate of the International Human Genome Authority (IHGA) to manage the human genome as the common heritage of mankind on behalf of all humanity is grounded, philosophically, in the ethics of responsible stewardship. The duties of stewardship towards the human genome should include protecting the genome from harm, such as the loss of genetic diversity or the propagation of harmful, human-induced mutations. Care must also be taken to avoid eugenics implications. It will be the duty of the IHGA to make sure that no one engages in forced sterilization, restricted procreation, ethnic cleansing, genocide, genetic discrimination or other immoral activities under the mistaken idea that we should purify the genome. Most people would agree that we have obligations not to engage in activities such as cloning and germ-line manipulation, if we determine that these activities pose a significant risk to future generations as well as a threat to the human gene pool. We must find some way of drawing a distinction between the obligation to avoid harming the human genome and the obligation to benefit the human genome. Although stewards normally have positive duties to benefit those things that they are entrusted with, there are sound moral reasons that suggest that these positive duties of stewardship should not extend to the human genome until we have a better understanding of the difference between therapy and enhancement in human genetics.

Duties of justice also demand that the IHGA manages the human genome justly and fairly. It will be the duty of the IHGA to ensure that current generations share the resources derived from the human genome with each other and with future generations. In doing so, the IHGA would be continuing where Arvid Pardo left off when at the age of 69, dismayed at the way the concept of common heritage of mankind was reduced in scope through the proceedings of the Law of the Sea Convention, he had predicted:

> [t]he present convention is not the end but rather the beginning of a long process that must eventually lead to a more rational and efficient use of our environment and a more equitable world order.[494]

---

[494] A. Pardo, *An Opportunity Lost*, quoted in Baslar, *The Concept of Common Heritage of Mankind in International Law* , p. 243.

The human genome is both the unalienable personal heritage of the individual and a fundamental component of the heritage of humanity and must therefore be protected. As time passes, we become increasingly capable of reading the characters and words in the DNA-book and this book is being opened wider with each day that passes.[495] At the same time, repositories holding human biological material such as national newborn screening-card collections or national pathology archives have been growing exponentially with hundreds of millions of samples that can be linked and converted into biobanks. Iceland and a few other countries have put together new collections of human material and associated health data from a representative part of the population. There has even been a proposal to set up a Global Biobank with the establishment of the Public Population Project in Genomics Consortium.[496] The fact that it will be possible to collect so much genomic data and connect it to health data on a global level leaves no doubt as to the wisdom of regulating the use of the human genome under the auspices of an international regime as the common heritage of mankind. The common heritage of mankind can form the philosophical basis for the global governance of the human genome in the shadow of technological progress that is a challenge to mankind in the deepest recesses of its humanity. International efforts to make a new international law for an acceptable and sustainable use of biotechnology are reflected in the Council of Europe Convention on Biomedicine (Oviedo Convention)[497] with its related Protocols on Human Cloning (1998),[498] the Transplantation of Organs and Tissues of Human Origin

---

[495]   Hans-Martin Sass, 'Why Protect the Human Genome', *Journal of Medicine and Philosophy*, 23:3(1998), 227–33.

[496]   J.A. Bovenberg, Inalienably Yours? The New Case for an Inalienable Property Right in Human Biological Material: Empowerment of Sample Donors or a Recipe for a Tragic Anti-Commons? (2004) 1:4 SCRIPT-ed 545. <http://www.law.ed.ac.uk/ahrb/script-ed/issue4/bovenberg.asp> [accessed on 20 January 2007]

[497]   Convention for the Protection of Human Rights and Dignity of the Human Being with Regard to the Application of Biology and Medicine: Convention on Human rights and Biomedicine, Oviedo, 4 April 1997, CETS n. 164.

[498]   Additional Protocol to the Convention for the Protection of Human Rights and Dignity of the Human Being with Regard to the Application of Biology and Medicine on the Prohibition of Cloning Human Beings, Paris, 12 January 1998, CETS n. 168.

$(2002)^{499}$ and Biomedical Research $(2005),^{500}$ together with the UNESCO Universal Declaration on the Human Genome $(1997)^{501}$ and the related Declaration on Human Genetic Data $(2003),^{502}$ the UN Declaration on Human Cloning $(2005)^{503}$ and the EC Directive on Biotechnological Inventions $(1998).^{504}$

Biotechnological developments continually pit conflicting principles against each other such as the free market patent system against the common heritage of mankind or the right to benefit from the advances in science and technology against the defense of human dignity and the integrity of the human person. As a philosophical concept, the common heritage of mankind can provide the space for continuing dialogue on issues of sovereignty, equitable justice and benefit-sharing aimed at working towards a foundation for biotechnology based on the human good. But lessons learnt from the past must not be forgotten lest we find ourselves in the same situation as Arvid Pardo, who, as the Law of the Sea Convention drew to a close, observed that, 'all that's left of the common heritage of mankind is a few fish and a little seaweed'.^{505}

We must not allow the concept of common heritage of mankind to be fossilized in its cradle as happened with the Law of the Sea Convention which practically encapsulated the concept in the potato-sized manganese nodules. Our task is to extract the DNA of the concept of common heritage of mankind and implant it in the human genome where it can grow to serve mankind. But the object of our study goes beyond this goal which can be readily achieved if the powers that be have the political will to do so. There is widespread concern that the science of the human genome is based upon a reductively biological perspective that is contrary to the meaning given to the human genome by the UNESCO General

---

[499] Additional Protocol to the Convention on Human rights and Biomedicine Concerning Transplantation of Organs and Tissues of Human Origin, Strasbourg, 24 January 2002, CETS n. 186.

[500] Additional Protocol to the Convention on Human rights and Biomedicine Concerning Biomedical Research, Strasbourg, 25 January 2005, CETS n. 195.

[501] Universal Declaration on the Human Genome and Human Rights, adopted by the General Conference of UNESCO at its 29th Session on 11 November 1997.

[502] International Declaration on Human Genetic Data, 16 October 2003.

[503] Declaration on Human Cloning, adopted by the General Assembly of the United Nations at its 59th Session on 8 March 2005.

[504] Directive 98/44/EC of the European Parliament and of the Council of 6 July 1998 on the Legal Protection of Biotechnological Inventions. OJL 213, 30 July 1998.

[505] Global Report, Center for War/Peace Studies 56 (1999/2000). <http://www.cwps.org /old/global56.htm> [accessed on 20 June 2007]

Conference Declaration on the Human Genome and Human Rights where in Article 1 the Declaration states that:

> The human genome underlies the fundamental unity of all members of the human family, as well as the recognition of their inherent dignity and diversity. In a symbolic sense, it is the heritage of humanity.[506]

This proclamation is considered the cornerstone of the Declaration with all provisions proceeding from the innovative nature of this notion. It will be the goal of the next stage of our study to explore the reasons why many biologists are dismissive of the importance of metaphysical considerations in discussing the human genome and why philosophers believe that one cannot discuss biological issues without metaphysical considerations.

---

[506]   Declaration on the Human Genome, Article 1.

Chapter Three
The Human Genome as Heritage of Humanity in a Symbolic Sense

3.1 Formatting the Genome

The human genome sequence has become central to ethical and policy debates on the application of genetic research to biomedicine and biotechnology. It is also shaping contemporary ideas about our *humanness* with scholars using the powerful scriptural metaphor of the 'Book of Man'[507] to refer to the human genome and likening its decoding to the search for the 'Holy Grail'.[508] Francis Crick, in his widely read book, '*Of Molecules and Men*', wrote:

> The ultimate aim of the modern movement in biology is in fact to explain **all** biology in terms of physics and chemistry.[509]

James Watson predicted that not only genetics but also other aspects of life are reducible to explanation at the molecular level:

> Complete certainty exists among essentially all biochemists that the other characteristics of living organisms (for example selective permeability across all membranes, muscle contraction and the hearing and memory process) will all be completely understood in terms of the coordinative interactions of large and small molecules.[510]

Before the HGP was even completed, Nobel Prize winner Walter Gilbert had enthusiastically announced that once the human genome was unraveled, mapped and sequenced, it would be possible to put together a sequence that represents the underlying structure of our humanity. Like many others before and after him, Gilbert was convinced that the secret of the Holy Grail would be revealed once the DNA-Book of Life was read from beginning to end! And like any other modern text, the DNA-Book could be burned on CDs. Gilbert predicted that it

---

[507] Bovenberg, *Property Rights in Blood, Genes and Data*, p. 11.
[508] Mauron, 'Is the Genome the Secular Equivalent of the Soul?', pp. 831–32.
[509] Francis Crick, *Of Molecules and Men* (New York: Prometheus Books, 1996), p. 10.
[510] James D. Watson, *The Molecular Biology of the Gene* (New York: 1966), p. 67.

would soon be possible to 'pull a CD out of one's pocket and say, "here is a human being; it's me"'.[511]

Gilbert's prediction very quickly became true when after the HGP was completed in April of 2003, Affymetrix Corporation was able to inscribe many of the hundreds of thousands of DNA sequences of the human genome on blue glass wafer microchips the size of a thumbnail. Affymetrix researchers are now able to rapidly scan gene sequences being expressed in the cells of living organisms and almost instantly determine the different DNA sequences in different genomes. The ultimate goal of this new biotechnology is the $1000 Genome when, for a fee of around $1000, by means of a small device, doctors would be able, from the comfort of their office, to read an individual's entire DNA sequencing code and in the process, identify any genetic disorders that may be present in the individual's genome.[512] Commenting on the $1000 Genome, Nicholas Wade from the *New York Times* wrote:

> When genomes can be decoded for $1000, a baby may arrive home like a new computer, with its complete genetic operating instructions on a DVD.[513]

In this section of our study, we shall examine the claims made by some authors that the secret of life is to be found in the text of the DNA-Book. We will demonstrate that this approach to the ontological nature of human life is based on a mistaken science that does not do justice to the essential nature of the human genome. This section has as its goal that of proving that the twin processes of making the human genome the common heritage of mankind and of overhauling the patent system with its focus on exclusive use rather than public use must be complemented with a science of the human genome that leaves no place for reductively biological considerations.

---

[511]   Richard M. Zaner, 'Surprise! You're Just Like Me! : Reflections on Cloning, Eugenics, and Other Utopias', in *Human Cloning*, ed. by James M. Humber and Robert F. Almeder (New Jersey: Humana Press, 1998), p. 105.

[512]   Ronald M. Green, *Babies by Design: The Ethics of Genetic Choice* (New Haven: Yale University Press, 2007), pp. 1–2.

[513]   Nicholas Wade, *The Quest for the $1,000 Human Genome*, quoted in Green, *Babies by Design*, p. 3.

3.2 Genes in a Test Tube?

Considering the benefits to mankind that the HGP promised to all those who could exploit it, the race to grab our DNA through the patenting system was inevitable. But when the first patent was issued way back in 1449 by King Henry VI to John of Utynam for a method of making stained glass with the proviso that the inventor must teach his art to others,[514] the situation was very different from what it is today where patents are being sought for human genes and academic research can be commercialized as a result of the *Bayh-Dole Act* of 1980.[515] Preoccupied that the patenting of human genes may lead to illegal profiteering from the human genome, several international bodies such as the United Nations Educational, Scientific, and Cultural Organization (UNESCO), the World Medical Association and the Human Genome Organization (HUGO) have all adopted specific statements about DNA patenting. While HUGO[516] declared that those who participate in genetic studies should receive some benefits from participation, both UNESCO and the World Medical Association[517] declared the human genome as the common heritage of mankind, and condemned any commercial benefit from the human genome in its natural state.[518] The World Medical Association even urged medical organizations around the world to lobby against gene patenting.[519]

The problem is that today the patenting system which sees the human genome as public property rather than common resource is supported by several scientists who choose to look upon the individual human being as nothing more than a 'combinatorial unit of re-assorted molecules'.[520] Metaphysically this is analogous to saying we are only DNA making more DNA. And when you reduce the individual to a 'combinatorial unit of re-assorted molecules', you are

---

[514] Resnik, *Owning the Genome*, p. 33.

[515] Bayh-Dole Act (The Patent and Trademark Law Amendments Act), enacted into law passed by the United States Congress on 12 December 1980. P.L. 96-517.

[516] Statement on Benefit-Sharing by the HUGO Ethics Committee, released on 9 April 2000.

[517] World Medical Association Declaration of Helsinki: Ethical Principles for Medical Research Involving Human Subjects, adopted by the 18th World Medical Association and amended by the 52nd WMA General Assembly, Edinburgh, Scotland, October 2000.

[518] Universal Declaration on the Human Genome and Human Rights, adopted by the General Conference of UNESCO at its 29th Session on 11 November 1997.

[519] World Medical Association Declaration of Helsinki (2000).

[520] David Holbrook (ed.), *What is it to be Human? New Perspectives in Philosophy* (Aldershot: Gower Publishing, 1990), p. 86.

in effect doing two things: on the one hand, reducing the individual to a complex entity made up of essentially non-living entities that have no moral value, and on the other hand, denying that the individual human being can be the subject of morality. The individual is divested of all moral value because morality only belongs to the living and when you consider the individual as a combination of non-living entities, there is no longer any place for moral conclusions.[521] The problem with this position is that it tends to deny the need to adopt a metaphysical account of human nature which is essential for addressing fundamental bioethical issues. Some bioethicists, in the empiricist tradition of David Hume, go so far as to deny that metaphysics can have any relevance to biomedical issues. This position is strongly contested by authors Philippa Foot,[522] Iris Murdoch[523] and others who believe that a metaphysical account of human nature is necessary to discuss ethical issues and therefore reject any form of reductionist thinking. It is unfortunate that there hasn't been a serious moral discussion between biologists who deny the relevance of metaphysics to biomedical issues and philosophers who hold that it is impossible to discuss these issues without metaphysical considerations.

Unfortunately, modern scientific thought has been taken over by a predominantly mechanistic understanding of Darwinism which rejects any form of teleological theory about the moral significance of the individual human being. It is an established fact that for many biologists today the chemical explanation of life and evolution has no need to resort to the idea of purpose or to what Aristotle termed final cause. Modern biology has no use for 'teleological' explanations—physico-chemical explanations are sufficient! According to Daniel C. Dennett, Darwin effectively put an end to any form of teleological thinking about the purpose and meaning of human life when he showed that the evolutionary process was the result of a mindless, algorithmic process which he termed 'natural selection'.[524] He compares Darwin's theory of natural selection to 'universal acid', a fantasy of his and some of his schoolboy friends, which is a liquid so

---

[521]   Ibid.

[522]   Philippa Foot has drawn upon the insights of Aquinas and Aristotle within the context of contemporary analytic philosophy. Her recent work has been seen by some as an attempt to modernize Aristotelian ethical theory.

[523]   Iris Murdoch's writings are a testimony to her lifelong project to retrieve a metaphysical framework for the moral life while at the same time defending the irreducibility of the individual.

[524]   Daniel C. Dennett, *Darwin's Dangerous Idea: Evolution and the Meanings of Life* (New York: Simon & Schuster, 1996), pp. 48–60.

corrosive that it practically dissolves anything which comes into contact with it![525] For Dennett, Darwin's theory of natural selection is such a universal acid because it has eaten through every traditional concept and has left in its wake a totally new world-view, in fact so new to Dennett, that he compares it to the Copernican Revolution:

> Darwin's dangerous idea is reductionism incarnate, promising to unite and explain just about everything in one magnificent vision. Its being the idea of an <u>algorithmic</u> process makes it all the more powerful, since the substrate neutrality it thereby possesses permits us to consider its application to just about anything. It is no respecter of material boundaries. It applies, as we have already begun to see, even to itself. The most common fear about Darwin's idea is that it will not just explain but <u>explain away</u> the Minds and Purposes and Meanings that we all hold dear. People fear that once this universal acid has passed through the monuments we cherish, they will cease to exist, dissolved in an unrecognizable and unlovable puddle of scientific destruction. This cannot be a sound fear; a proper reductionistic explanation of these phenomena would leave them still standing but just demystified, unified, placed on more secure foundations.[526]

This position is very contrary to that of several contemporary philosophers who are beginning to think of the human genome as embodying our humanness, determining both our individuality and our species-identity. This genomic metaphysics sees the genome as being the true essence of human nature with external influences considered as accidental events. This notion of the human genome is very similar to the Aristotelian notion of *eidos* which is the organizing principle inherent in every living thing. Aristotle and Aquinas saw *eidos* as closely connected to the notion of soul which gave a living organism its distinguishing characteristics as well as the essence of the organism's species. For Aristotle, it was not only human beings who had a soul but so did plants and animals with a vegetative and sensitive soul respectively.[527]

With the human embryo denied its moral status or *forma* as the embodiment of our species-identity and personal identity and reduced to a 'blob of cells' or a 'conglomeration of molecules',[528] the slippery slope to the patenting and commercialization of the human genome was inevitable. Richard Dawkins, com-

---

[525] Dennett goes so far as to deny teleonomy, i.e., that there is some apparent purposefulness and goal-directedness in the structures and functions of living organisms that are derived from their evolutionary history and adaptation for reproductive success.

[526] Ibid., p. 82.

[527] Mauron, 'Is the Genome the Secular Equivalent of the Soul?', pp. 831–32.

[528] Holbrook, 'Medical Ethics and the Potentialities of the Living Being', pp. 459–62 (p. 459).

menting on Darwin's theory of natural selection, explains that the theory is satisfying because it shows a way how simplicity could change into complexity when unordered atoms group themselves into more complex molecules until they end up manufacturing people. On the same lines, Paul Atkins, in his book *Creation*, wrote:

> I shall take your mind on a journey. It is a journey. It is a journey of comprehension, taking us to the edge of space, time and understanding. On it I shall argue that there is nothing that cannot be understood, that there is nothing that cannot be explained, and that everything is extraordinarily simple...A great deal of the universe does not need any explanation. Elephants, for instance, once molecules have learnt to compete and to create other molecules in their own image, elephants and things resembling elephants, will in due course be found roaming through the countryside.[529]

According to Dawkins, Darwin provides the only feasible solution to the deep problem of man's existence. It stands to reason that this position not only undermines the consideration that the human genome constitutes the distinctive element that is specific to each individual as a component of his or her uniqueness but also undermines the consideration that the human genome should not be made the object of appropriation as it is a 'common resource'.

3.3   Darwin Revisited!

But the crux of the matter is that Darwin's theory of natural selection and Aristotle's teleological approach to human nature are not mutually exclusive. According to Leon Kass, there is no problem in reconciling Darwin's theory of natural selection with an understanding of organisms as purposive beings.[530] According to him, the problem lies in a mistaken interpretation of teleology. To explain his point he makes two interesting observations, the first on a letter which Asa Gray sent to his friend Darwin in 1874 and the second on Darwin's reply to Gray's letter. In his letter to Darwin, Asa Gray, himself a renowned botanist and evolutionist, wrote:

---

[529]   Peter Atkins, *The Creation*, quoted in Richard Dawkins, *The Blind Watchmaker: Why the Evidence of Evolution Reveals a Universe Without Design* (New York: W.W. Norton & Company, 1986), p. 14.

[530]   Leon Kass was Chairman of the President's Council on Bioethics from 2001 to 2005.

> Let us recognize Darwin's great service to Natural Science in bringing back to it teleology; so that, instead of Morphology versus Teleology, we shall have Morphology wedded to Teleology.[531]

To this, Darwin replied:

> What you say about Teleology pleases me especially, and I do not think any one else has ever noticed the point.[532]

In a word, Darwin never meant to reject all teleological ideas about life and nature. For Leon Kass, Darwinism cannot be correctly understood without the notion of teleology. The root of the problem lies with the tendency of the modern mind to appropriate science and the scientific method for its own anti-metaphysical ends, thus reducing rational analysis to reductionism with its inherent skepticism. On these lines, Victor Frankl, in an essay on *Reductionism and Nihilism*, had written:

> Reductionism is more than just saying time and again that something is nothing but something else. It is an approach and procedure that deprives the human phenomena of their very humanness by reducing a human phenomenon in dynamic terms to some sub-human phenomenon, or deducing human phenomena, in genetic terms, from sub-human phenomena.[533]

When one is able to go beyond the reductionist approach to natural science, it becomes evident, from an accurate reading of Darwin's *The Origin of the Species*, that in explaining natural selection, Darwin was in fact mainly concerned with explaining the teleological character of living organisms. In his introduction to '*The Origin of the Species*', Darwin wrote:

> In considering the Origin of Species, it is quite conceivable that a naturalist, reflecting on the mutual affinities of organic beings, on their embryological relations, their geographical distribution, geological succession, and other such facts, might come to the conclusion that species had not been independently created, but had descended, like varieties, from other species.

---

[531]   Leon R. Kass, *Toward a More Natural Science: Biology and Human Affairs* (New York: The Free Press, 1988), p. 252.

[532]   Ibid.

[533]   V.E. Frankl, 'Reductionism and Nihilism', in *Beyond Reductionism: New Perspectives in the Life Sciences,* ed. by A. Koestler and J.R. Smythies (London: Hutchinson, 1969), p. 402.

Nevertheless, such a conclusion, even if well founded, would be unsatisfactory, until it could be shown how the innumerable species inhabiting this world have been modified, so as to acquire that perfection of structure and coadaptation which justly excites our admiration.[534]

Therefore, Darwin was interested in explaining not only the internal purposiveness which was to be found in plants and animals but also the underlying reason for the perfection which he could observe not only in their structure but also in the ordered set of relations which governed their activity as members of the same kind.

Though offspring often resemble their parents, variations occur in all parts of an organism, which variations can be transmitted to the progeny of the organism carrying the variations. And, as species reproduce at a much faster rate than they are able to replenish their food resources, the excess of offspring in relation of the food available results in the survival of only those organisms that undergo variations that give them an advantage over the other members of the species. This is Darwin's natural selection, basically the survival of organisms with advantageous variations, the consequent transmission of these heritable traits to their offspring, and the elimination of deleterious traits as the most unfit organisms fail to survive. The principle of natural selection is therefore based on two factors, both related to change, namely the origin of novelty and the preservation of novelty. In a nutshell, the variation responsible for the appearance of novelty and the process of natural selection proper ensure that this novelty is preserved by being transmitted to the progeny of the organisms that are carriers of these novel variations.

There are two important implications of this integrative rather than reductionist approach to Darwin's theory of natural selection. The first is that Darwin succeeds in giving a non-teleological account of the origin of and basis for the teleological character of organisms by demonstrating that purposive and co-adapted beings and races rise and change and fall by processes that are themselves not purposive and out of a nature that is seemingly purposeless and aimless. At the same time, and this brings us to the second implication of Darwin's theory, his non-teleological explanation of natural selection, comprising variation, inheritance, and struggle for existence, depends upon the immanent teleological character of organisms, a fact which Darwin appears to take for granted.

In respect of this immanent teleological aspect of life, evolutionary biologists today are apprehensive of the fact that the central ethical question about

---

[534]   Charles Darwin, *The Origin of Species: By Means of Natural Selection* (Middlesex: Senate, 1998), p. 2.

the passage from conception to birth remains focused on the issue of 'When does life begin?'. From an evolutionary biologist's point of view, the question is very easy to answer because 'life began 3.5 billion years ago and has existed continuously ever since!' Stephen J. Gould wrote in his book, *I have landed: The end of a beginning in natural history*:

> ...I would nominate as most worthy of pure awe—a metaphorical miracle, if you will—an aspect of life that most people have never considered, but that strikes me as equal in majesty to our most spiritual projections of infinity and eternity, while falling entirely within the domain of our conceptual and empirical grasp: the continuity of *etz chayim*, the tree of earthly life, for at least 3.5 billion years, without a single microsecond of disruption.[535]

The fact that all beings alive today are linked by an unbroken chain of life that extends billions of years into the past has many ethical and philosophical implications and it is no wonder that many evolutionary biologists have felt a sense of wonder and awe at this evolutionary insight. By his theory of natural selection, Darwin explained the essential connection that exists between the desire to be found in living organisms to survive and propagate and the teleological nature of these organisms. In other words, it is the teleological nature of life that provides the *nexus* between natural selection and the miracle of the continuity of life—at the heart of natural selection is the teleological nature of these organisms—these organisms survive because they are teleological! This is not to say that these organisms are teleological because they survived—this is the teleological interpretation of Darwin's thought that Dawkins and others never tire of attacking. In expounding his theory of natural selection, Darwin reaffirmed the teleological force of nature which is at the heart of the natural process of evolution.[536]

Marjorie Greene, commenting on those biologists who adamantly refuse to accept the goal-centeredness which was so evident in the biological world, wrote:

> The theoretical framework of the biologist's training is centred—implicitly and indirectly if not explicitly and directly—in the theory of evolution by Mendelian micromutations and natural selection. In terms of ultimate beliefs, this means the view that the present population of the earth's surface is derived by a repetition of a few simple mechanisms...from unicellular and ultimately from non-living particles of matter. This picture is associated also with an aggregative conception of the organism itself. 'Ultimately', one believes an organism such as a

---

[535]   Stephen J. Gould, *I Have Landed: The End of a Beginning in Natural History* (New York: Harmony Books, 2002), p. 14.

[536]   Kass, *Toward a More Natural Science*, 1988, pp. 260–61.

mouse or a frog or a man will be identifiable in terms of material particles and their spatio-temporal relationships...The trained biologist, in other words, works under the aegis of a guiding principle that organisms are aggregates of material particles moved by mechanical, physico-chemical laws...Scientific discourse, accordingly, qua scientific must be wholly non- and anti-teleological, and any speech tainted with teleology must remain wholly extraneous to science.[537]

Greene is harsh in her condemnation of those scientists who reject outright any teleological goal in biological life, including human life. But her reaction is understandable when one ponders for a minute what we stand to lose, as human beings, if we allow this way of doing science to dominate the field of biotechnology when we are at the advent of a new genetic age. As Professor Marjorie Greene[538] has pointed out, to many philosophical biologists, especially those trained in the atmosphere of British science, only that which is non-living is real, because only what is non-living can be explained in terms of molecules. This mode of thinking is not concerned with Being, the autonomous, dynamic organization and potentiality of the living creature because it cannot explain it!

Michael Polanyi remarks that while teleology has become a dirty word for us,[539] this was not always the case. Before modern science interpreted Darwin's evolutionary theory in a predominantly mechanistic way, there was no opposition to teleological thoughts about man and nature. Not only was man seen to have a special purpose or function but even other living things, with their specific integrative structure of organs and tissues.

All this changed with modern science's mechanistic interpretation of Darwin's origin of the species and modern biology's attempts to explain life processes in terms of chemical and physical mechanisms.

Polanyi believes that the major obstacle to the possibility of entertaining any sort of teleological views is the reduction of life processes to physical and chemical laws. Although in a given DNA molecule there is a finite number of physical and chemical mechanisms, still, argues Polanyi, we cannot explain and identify with accuracy these mechanisms and therefore, the reduction of life processes into physical and chemical laws is, to say the least, premature. Completely chemical and physical explanations for certain crucial aspects of living

---

[537]   Marjorie Grene, 'Time and Teleology', in *The Knower and the Known*, ed. by Marjorie Grene (New York: Basic Books, 1966), pp. 234–35.

[538]   Marjorie Grene, 'The Faith of Darwinism', in *The Knower and the Known* (New York: Basic Books, 1966), p. 185.

[539]   Polanyi and Prosch, *Meaning*, p. 163.

things have not been found, in spite of the momentous discovery of DNA.[540] Although it has generally been assumed that since organisms are mechanisms and since mechanisms work in accordance with physical and chemical laws, organisms must also work in the same way, biological mechanisms cannot be explained as the resultants of the operation of physical and chemical laws only. This is because there are two aspects of a biological mechanism that must be taken into account and these are (i) the factual aspect comprising the physical and chemical conditions which permit the physical and chemical reactions specific to the particular mechanism to take place and (ii) the boundary conditions or limits within which the particular physical and chemical reactions take place. These boundary conditions, for Polanyi, determine the pattern in which these physical and chemical interactions are put together rather than the way in which these physical and chemical parts interact with one another. For Polanyi, though all living organisms appear to function in a way that appears to be guided by meaningful boundary conditions, a mechanism acquires its organization by reference to some aim or goal or purpose that is to be achieved by it and this purpose cannot be deduced from the physico-chemical aspect of the mechanism.[541] The same applies to all living organisms and in fact, Polanyi observes,

> This is not to deny that there is a great deal of truth in the mechanical explanation of life. The organs of the body work much like machines, and they are subject to a hierarchy of controls, exercised by an ascending series of mechanical principles. Biologists pursuing the aim of explaining living functions in terms of machines have achieved astounding success. But this must not obscure the fact that these advances only add to the features of life which cannot be represented in terms of laws manifested in the realm of inanimate nature.[542]

Just as the intelligent sequencing of the dots and dashes in Morse code require a higher principle to create a meaningful message, likewise the genetic information carried by the DNA which guides the development and functioning of a living organism requires a higher level of control that transcends the material laws of physics and chemistry. This is why physical biologists are wrong when they suggest that the DNA functions as a code for the chemical and physical development of the organism. It is an undisputed fact that a necessary feature of a code is that it must be chemically and physically neutral to the messages if it is to transmit them. For example, it is because ink blobs do not have a physical

---

[540] Polanyi and Prosch, *Meaning*, p. 167.
[541] Polanyi, 'Life Transcending Physics and Chemistry', pp. 54–66.
[542] Polanyi, *The Tacit Dimension*, p. 42.

or chemical reaction with paper that they can be used as part of a linguistic system to communicate meaningful messages such as the ideas in this thesis. Furthermore, it is precisely because the ink blobs are part of a linguistic system and so do not appear on paper as the mere result of random equilibrations of forces, that they are able to convey meaningful messages.

In other words, the dynamics of a living cell cannot be explained by reduction to the laws governing DNA molecules because in the molecules of life there is a fantastic configuration of forms and activities which require being studied in yet another dimension. While the shaping of the boundaries which are represented by the physical-chemical forms establishes a 'controlling principle', the system itself is put under the control of a non-physical-chemical principle by a 'profoundly informative intervention'.[543] Polanyi believes that life is characterized by a 'striving forward' which can be explained as a 'gradient' towards higher forms and self-consciousness. The high level of genetic possibilities in man as compared with a lower animal is a manifestation of this striving, and each individual, as it comes into being, is a fresh manifestation of the attempt by life to develop potentialities. As Polanyi points out, the apparent simplicity of the chemical composition of the DNA molecule masks the complexity of the process involved in the generation of new life and the qualitative progression in the evolution of the species and the generation of life within the same species.

> How can we account for the transmission of life from one generation to the next? A fertilized egg will develop into an organized system including thousands of millions of new cells in the modified image of its ancestors. The successive stages of the embryo are each larger than its immediate precursor, each more differentiated and all these transformations are accomplished by the division of existing arrays of cells into twice as many new cells.[544]

Each step in this expansion is induced by the surroundings of the DNA compounds at that stage and these guiding surroundings are due to the guiding surroundings of a previous stage and so on. In other words, each stage of the biological growth anticipates the subsequent step of growth by producing for its guidance a cellular body, which will instruct the cellular divisions of the next stage and will carry on the development to the final product.

Polanyi, like many others, makes the mistake of comparing the role of the DNA as a guide to the physiological development of the foetus to an architectural blueprint used to guide the building of a new edifice. The blueprint analogy

---

[543]   Polanyi, *Life Transcending Physics and Chemistry*, pp. 54–66.
[544]   Polanyi and Prosch, *Meaning*, p. 165.

fails because while the blueprint is merely a guide for the builder to know how to proceed, step by step, in his endeavor to complete the project he is working on, the DNA molecule is both the builder and the blueprint and it knows how to act differently, at different times in the different stages of the development of the foetus. This foetal development is characterized by three key words, coordination, continuity and gradualness. It is a miracle of nature how the foetus develops from one cell to a fully developed baby. It is in this respect that the analogy with of the DNA with an architectural blueprint fails. Whereas in the latter case it is the architect who is the mind behind the blueprint, the DNA is itself the mind and the blueprint. In guiding the successive stages of the embryonic development, the DNA is responsible for producing a sequence of cellular milieu(s) associated with different actions of the same DNA in order to bring to termination the development of the embryo.[545] It stands to reason that for the DNA to function in this manner its role within the dynamics of embryonic development cannot be reduced to that of a chemical compound that merely responds chemically to other chemical compounds in the human body. A more plausible explanation would be that the DNA is a 'master molecule', that is at once the blueprint and the architect's mind and is able to act in a purposeful way (something that cannot be explained in purely chemical way) or else the DNA is another 'organ' in the body that is able to interrelate with the other organs by 'adapting' to the specific needs of the particular organism in question for growth and maintenance.[546]

Many biologists like Erwin Schrödinger who have pointed to the need to take into account the dimensions of activities in living creatures have not as yet, as it is often declared, found the secret of life, for large areas of that secret are still mysterious and unfathomable. In his book, *What is life?* Schrödinger describes the structural and thermodynamic properties which are the characteristic of the molecules of living cells. The entire complex of terrestrial life is based on chains of the same four DNA compounds with each organism having its own distinctive sequence of them. The genetic code is the same for all living organisms from bacteria to humans. The constitutive mechanism of the system permits an infinite possibility of permutations like those with the letters of the alphabet. The DNA chain of a bacterium carries about 20 million alterations, that of an insect around 200 million and those of a human being about 12 billion.

---

[545]   Michael and Prosch, *Meaning*, p. 166.
[546]   Ibid., pp. 166–67.

The constitutive mechanism of the genetic code allows this quantitative increase in DNA as we proceed along the evolutionary ladder.[547] Erwin Schrödinger wrote:

> ...the chromosomes...contain, in some kind of codified script, the entire pattern of the individual's future development and of his functioning in the mature state. Every complete set of chromosomes contains the full code.[548]

Schrödinger argued that life could be thought of in terms of storing and passing on biological information. Chromosomes were thus simply information bearers. Because so much information had to be passed in every cell, it must be compressed into what Schrödinger called a 'hereditary code-script' embedded in the molecular fabric of chromosomes. According to Schrödinger, although the identification of these molecules and the cracking of their code would lead us closer to understanding life, the true meaning of it was to be found beyond the laws of physics.[549] Talking about Galilean principles or the laws of physics, Charles Taylor writes:

> But to assume from the superiority of Galilean principles in the sciences of inanimate nature that they must provide the model for the sciences of animate behaviour is to make a speculative leap, not to enunciate a necessary conclusion.[550]

These metaphysical reflections on the human genome can never be reconciled with the patenting of human genes which makes parts of the human genome subject to appropriation by individuals and groups through the granting of intellectual property rights. As has been demonstrated, the human genome is not a collection of genes that can be explored and exploited but rather, the human genome is a metaphysical reality that defies the method of scientific control. It was mainly for this reason that the drafters of the Universal Declaration on the Human Genome and Human Rights chose, after long deliberation to refer to the

---

[547]   Watson, *DNA: The Secret of Life*, pp. 36–37.
[548]   Schrödinger, *What is Life?*, p. 21.
[549]   Watson, *DNA: The Secret of Life*, p. 35.
[550]   Charles Taylor, *The Explanation of Behaviour* (London: Routledge & Kegan Paul, 1980), p. 25.

human genome as being the heritage of humanity, 'in a symbolic sense',[551] rather than simply, the 'common heritage of humanity'.[552] The second version was adopted because of fears that the first version might lead to a reductionist approach to the human genome that would reduce it to a collection of human genes that could be patented and so be made subject to the restrictions normally imposed through the granting of exclusive intellectual property rights. The adoption of the second version also raises questions about the legitimacy of patenting human genes when as such these genes are not being invented but rather simply discovered! And even the question of discovery raises questions of concern since these genes have existed for many and many years and so, as common heritage of humanity, should remain free from appropriation by any individual or group. It is illogical to argue in favour of the granting of exclusive intellectual property rights on human genes that belong to me as much as they belong to you!

3.4 The Genie in the Genome

Teilhard de Chardin arrives to the same conclusion about the teleological nature of life but from a different perspective that looks upon the *secret of life* from an evolutionary angle. Like many contemporary scientists, he was convinced that evolution involved the development of higher forms of life from lower ones that came before. Not only, but the human species was also the most highly developed of all natural species. Like Teilhard, many scientists today believe that the human being has evolved from lower class mammals over eons of time and they in turn were generated from even lower forms, back to the simplest forms of life. Scientifically speaking, this generation of one life form from and to another can only take place as a result of changes in genetic properties in the course of time. Making a distinction between the 'within' and 'without' of things, Teilhard remarks that the physicist is mainly concerned with the 'without' of things:

> ...objects in the realm of physico-chemistry are only made manifest by their outward determinisms... In the eyes of the physicist, nothing exists legitimately, at least up to now, except

---

[551] Universal Declaration on the Human Genome and Human Rights, adopted by the General Conference of UNESCO at its 29th Session on 11 November 1997, Article 1.

[552] UNESCO, *Birth of the Universal Declaration on the Human Genome and Human Rights* (Paris: UNESCO, 1999), p. 1.

the without of things. The same intellectual attitude is still permissible in the bacteriologist, whose cultures (apart from some substantial difficulties) are treated as laboratory reagents.[553]

But, according to Teilhard, the unity to be found on the level of the 'without' must be complemented on the level of the 'within':

> In everything, therefore, Teilhard distinguishes a double aspect: an exterior, which relates only to the observable connections and dimensions of material things, and an interior—an interior aspect of things which is to be envisaged as co-extensive with their exterior and in some degree is present in them all.[554]

For Teilhard, this complementarity between the 'without' and 'within' becomes apparent with the arrival of man on the evolutionary landscape.[555] In fact, he argues that the intellectual attitude which refuses to acknowledge this 'interiority' of the world of existence becomes very difficult to sustain when studying the behaviour of insects or coelenterates, futile when studying vertebrates and totally meaningless when studying man!

> From a purely positivist point of view man is the most mysterious and disconcerting of all objects met with by science. In fact we may as well admit that science has not yet found a place for him in its representations of the universe. Physics has succeeded in provisionally circumscribing the world of the atom. Biology has been able to impose some sort of order on the constructions of life. Supported both by physics and biology, anthropology in its turn does its best to explain the structure of the human body and some of its physiological mechanisms. But when all these features are put together, the portrait manifestly falls short of the reality.[556]

At the same time, as science is able to make a more precise and penetrating study of the facts of nature, and the more man is able to penetrate into matter by means of increasingly powerful methods, the more we find ourselves confounded by the interdependence of its parts! For Teilhard, the universe can only be taken as a whole, as one piece, where each element of the cosmos is interwoven with the

---

[553] Teilhard De Chardin, *The Phenomenon of Man*, trans. by Bernard Hall (New York: Harper & Row Publishers, 1975), p. 55.

[554] N.M. Wildiers, *Teilhard de Chardin* (London: William Collins sons & Co., 1969), p. 78.

[555] Teilhard tried to go beyond the Cartesian duality of Mind and Matter but in doing so he appeared to enforce the Cartesan model if not even extend it by using the Within and Without (Spirit and Matter) distinction in terms of two energies. It would have been better if he had spoken in Einsteinian terms of conversion of energy. Teilhard did not mean to make the mistake and in fact his ideas could easily be reformulated from this perspective that bypasses the Cartesian model.

[556] Ibid., p. 163.

other elements and it is impossible to cut into this network, to isolate a portion, without it becoming frayed and unraveled at all its edges.

The same can be said of the DNA chain. The parts making up the chain do not have to be arranged chemically in the manner in which they are in order for the chain to function as a medium for message transmission. Each item of a DNA series is made up of one of four alternative organic bases which, in turn, have equal probability of forming any particular item in the series. It is on the basis of this equal probability of all the four bases to form any particular item in the DNA series that the DNA can effectively function as a code. If the DNA were an ordinary chemical molecule, it would not be able to function as a code because its chemical structure would be due to its having achieved maximum stability and this chemical orderliness would prevent it from functioning as a code.

Therefore, every living organism is a meaningful organization of meaningless matter and it is very highly improbable that these meaningful organizations could have all occurred by chance. Furthermore, it would appear to us that the general trend in the evolutionary development of living organisms has been towards more meaningful organizations, both in their constitutive organizational structure and in their capacity to communicate meaningfully with other beings:

> From microscopic one-celled plants, able to do very little more than to provide for their own sustenance and to reproduce, to minute animals, sensitive as individuals to their surroundings and able to learn very rudimentary sustaining habits, to more complex animals, able to do many more things, to the higher mammals and finally to man, who is able to achieve so many things that he frequently supposes himself to be a god able to achieve all things—man's evolutionary history is a panorama of meaningful achievements of almost breathtaking proportions. And when one considers, in the face of the staggering number of merely chemical possibilities open to DNA that so many meaningful combinations have come into existence and that these have been oriented in the direction of the achievement of more and more meaning (even when change in this direction did not always relate to the necessities of survival), it is difficult to avoid the notions that some sort of gradient of meaning is operative in evolution in addition to purely accidental molecular and plain natural selection and that this gradient somehow evokes even more meaningful organization (i.e. boundary conditions) of matter.[557]

Teilhard believed that evolution was a purposeful process which would reach a climax at some point in the future, where this point represented a kind of totally integrated state of life. For him, this point was the Omega point, the point which the universe is destined to reach. To him, those scientists who propounded the

---

[557] Polanyi and Prosch, *Meaning*, p. 173.

myth that we are mere bystanders on a speck of dust far from the heart of the Universe were doing the *phenomena of life* a disservice.[558]

Teilhard de Chardin, concerned with the metaphysical and ethical implications of this reductionist position on human life, gives a wonderful interpretation of the value of human life and evolution in his book, *The Phenomenon of Life*:

> The time has come to realize that an interpretation of the universe—even a positivist one—remains unsatisfying unless it covers the interior as well as the exterior of things: mind as well as matter. The true physics is that which will, one day, achieve the inclusion of man in his wholesome in a coherent picture of the world.[559]

The truth of the matter is that the emergence of life, especially of mind, are mysteries which we cannot explain and it is very unlikely that they came into existence simply as a result of the collision of matter. If we take the process of development of the embryo as an example, we soon realize that it involves a complex sequence of relative cell movements which cannot be reduced to the mechanism of mere chance and necessity. Even a simple protozoon, a hundredth of an inch long, moving at 600 micrometers a minute, exhibits behaviour and autonomy which mechanism cannot explain.

With the work of Teilhard de Chardin it is not difficult to comprehend the importance of safe-guarding the human genome as a common heritage of mankind for and on behalf of all humanity. The human genome is both the unalienable personal heritage of the individual and a fundamental component of the heritage of humanity and must therefore be protected. This means that any biotechnological interventions that crossed the line between the 'within' and 'without' of the human genome had to be banned because they threatened the fundamental essence of our humanness that embodies both our individual identity and the identity of our species.

3.5   The Transcendental Nature of the Human Genome

Michael Polanyi and Teilhard de Chardin have shown in their writings that the teleology that modern science rejects is nothing less than 'an overriding cosmic purpose necessitating all the structures and occurrences in the universe to accomplish itself'.[560] Both Polanyi and Teilhard share the conviction that the

---

[558]   Teilhard de Chardin, *The Vision of the Past*, trans. by J.M. Cohen (London: Collins 1966), pp. 52–52.

[559]   De Chardin, *The Phenomenon of Man*, pp. 35–36.

[560]   Polanyi and Prosch, *Meaning*, p. 162.

world is thought to be absurd by modern man not because there is no order in the universe but rather because there is no particular purpose to it. Teilhard, who was called a loser by Daniel Dennett in his book *Darwin's Dangerous Idea* because he denied that evolution was a mindless, purposeless, algorithmic process, sought a science that was concerned with the totality of the cosmic phenomenon and which sought to probe right into its structure and inner dynamism. Naturally, this science had to be aided by all other sciences with all they had achieved in their respective fields. But, at the same time, this science had to embrace and transcend all other sciences and focus only on what is most specifically of the whole:

> We must not lose sight of the fact that the whole is more than the sum of its constituent parts. A plant is more than the sum of the chemical elements occurring in it. The world too is more than the sum of the entities found in it; and because that is so, it is not enough just to combine the results obtained from the various natural sciences in order to arrive at a true picture of what the world really is.[561]

Polanyi rejects the idea that the universe and all it contains, including us humans, is simply the product of purely material processes and events. But unlike William Paley[562] who pictured God as making the universe like a 'watch', Polanyi attributed design to an evolutionary process which is not personified and which cannot be described in the scientific language of physics and chemistry.[563] Although this kind of teleology appears to be a form of determinism which rejects a radical freedom on the part of human beings, Polanyi argues for a loose view of teleology that permits him to postulate in favour of some sort of intelligible directional tendency operative in the world, without having to suppose that this directional tendency determines all things.

This philosophical thinking, rather than arguing in favour of determinism of purpose, proposes a 'theory of forces' in the sense that the tendency towards achievement of more meaningful or orderly or regular relations is inexplicable unless there is some directional force, immanent and operative in all living things.

In *The Future of Man*, Teilhard writes:

---

[561] Wildiers, *Teilhard de Chardin*, p. 48.
[562] Dawkins, *The Blind Watchmaker*, 1996, pp. 1–18.
[563] Michael Polanyi, *Personal knowledge: Towards a Post-Critical Philosophy* (London: Routledge, 2002), p. 390.

> Let us suppose that from this universal centre, this Omega point, there constantly emanate radiations hitherto only perceptible to those persons whom we call 'mystics'. Let us further imagine that, as the sensibility or response to mysticism of the human race increases with planetisation, the awareness of Omega becomes so widespread as to warm the earth psychically while physically it is growing cold. Is it not conceivable that Mankind, at the end of its totalisation, its folding-in upon itself, may reach a critical level of maturity where, leaving Earth and stars to lapse slowly back into dwindling mass of primordial energy, it will detach itself from this planet and join the one true, irreversible essence of things, the Omega point?[564]

Teilhard portrayed the cosmos as energy in the process of evolutionary movement towards greater systems of complexity, involving three critical points marked by profound changes:

1) the emergence of inorganic matter;
2) the appearance of life and the growth of the biosphere and,
3) the appearance of mind and humanity.

With regards to the third stage, Teilhard maintained that evolution could follow a conscious direction. He believed that evolution maintained a definite direction or 'Ariadne's Thread', as he called it. The thread was the increasing complexity of living beings, with the focus on the nervous systems, especially the brains.[565] This progressive complexification was manifested in the world of nature by the emergence, over time, of living beings with an ever greater capacity for communication. If one compares a fish to an ape, for example, it is obvious that evolution moves towards a maximization of communicative abilities.

For this reason, Teilhard uses words like 'noogenesis' to mean the gradual evolution of mind as mental properties and repeatedly stresses that we should no longer speak of a cosmology but of a 'cosmogenesis'. Similarly, he likes to use a pregnant term like 'hominization' to denote the process by which the original proto-human stock became, and is still becoming, more truly human and the process by which potential man revealed more and more of his possibilities. Indeed he extends this evolutionary terminology by employing terms like 'ultra-hominization' to denote the deducible future stage of the process in which man will have so far transcended himself as to demand some new appellation.

To Teilhard, the future was to be characterized by a progressive extension of higher consciousness which would not only increase the process of individualization and personal freedom but also proceed towards greater communion and

---

[564]   Teilhard de Chardin, *The Future of Man,* trans. by Norman Denny (New York: Doubleday, 2004), pp. 115–16.
[565]   De Chardin, *Phenomenon of Man*, p. 142.

socialization on a planetary scale. Finally, there would be a convergence of humanity towards what he called the Omega point when the process of evolution will reach its culmination in a suprapersonal unity in God in which self-transcending love would rule all.

With this approach he is rightly and indeed inevitably driven to the conclusion that, since evolutionary phenomena, including the phenomenon known as Man, are processes, they can never be evaluated or even adequately described solely or mainly in terms of their origins—they must be defined by their direction, their inherent possibilities, including of course also their terminations, and their deducible future trends. He quotes with approval Nietzsche's view that man is unfinished and must be surpassed or completed; and proceeds to deduce the steps needed for his completion.[566]

For Teilhard, a developed human being is not merely a more highly individualized individual. He has crossed the threshold of self-consciousness to a new mode of thought and as a result has achieved some degree of conscious integration—the integration of the self with the outer world of men and nature and the integration of the separate elements of the self with each other. He is a person, an organism, which has transcended individuality in personality. This attainment of personality was an essential element in man's past and present evolutionary success: accordingly its fuller achievement must be an essential aim for his evolutionary future.

When one considers Teilhard's thoughts on evolution, we are left with no doubt with regards to our responsibilities towards future generations. Filled with 'totally human hope',[567] Teilhard believes that there is no room for complacency because mankind is consciously becoming aware of its shortcomings and its capacities and therefore is ready to shoulder its responsibilities:

> ...the power acquired by a consciousness to turn in upon itself, to take possession of itself as of an object endowed with its own particular consistence and value: no longer merely to know, but to know oneself; no longer merely to know but to know that one knows. By this individualization of himself in the depths of himself, the living element, which heretofore had been spread out and divided over a diffuse circle of perceptions and activities, was constituted for the first time as a centre in the form of a point at which all the impressions and experiences knit themselves together and fuse into a unity that is conscious of its own organization.[568]

---

[566]   De Chardin, *Future of Man*, p. 133.
[567]   Teilhard de Chardin, *The Divine Milieu* (New York: Perennial, 2001), p. 132.
[568]   De Chardin, *Phenomenon of Man*, p. 165.

Teilhard's understanding of evolution is of pivotal importance in comprehending the vital connection between the HGP and future generations.[569] His universe was one of continuous and interwoven evolutionary threads, incorporating plants, animals, the planets, the cosmos and the physical and mental evolution of mankind. Michael Murray, in his book, *The Thought of Teilhard de Chardin*, writes:

> Man [is] the growing tip of the evolutionary axis—man, the most complex and conscious entity so far produced by the universe as a whole. Physically small, but psychically the superlative result of all synthetic labours of the stars, man is the spiritual, if not the spatial summit of the cosmos, the hope and instrument of its future consummation. Thus in Teilhard's hands the theory of evolution, far from diminishing man by relating him to the apes, as so many churchmen used to fear, actually re-establishes him at the moving apex of time-space, well above the fixed central position which he lost in the Copernican revolution.[570]

Evolution, for Teilhard, is characterized by 'convergence' or 'integration'. The most important evolutionary leap was the formation of the 'noosphere', which, as Michael Murray explains, begins with,

> ...a global network of trade, communications, accumulation and exchange of knowledge, co-operative research, mixture of populations and production of energy—all go into the weaving of the material support for a sphere of collective thought. In the field of science alone, no individual knows more than a tiny fraction of the sum of scientific knowledge, and each scientist is dependent not only for his education but for all his subsequent work on the traditions and resources which are the collective possession of an entire international society composed of the living and the dead. Just as Earth once covered itself with a film of interdependent living organisms which we call the biosphere, so mankind's combined achievements are forming a global network of collective mind.[571]

Man, for Teilhard, is not the random product of evolution. To him the process of evolution is planned and guided. Together with Paley, Teilhard is a firm believer of the presence of a 'watchmaker' who makes things work. It is therefore not surprising that Richard Dawkins and other militant atheists chose to ridicule and accuse Teilhard of obscurantism.[572] One may in fact consider Dawkins' book, the *Blind Watchmaker*, as a total rejection of Teilhard's thoughts. But

---

[569]   Teilhard de Chardin, *Building the Earth* (London: Geoffrey Chapman, 1965), pp. 75–77.
[570]   Michael H. Murray, *The Thought of Teilhard de Chardin* (New York: Seabury Press, 1966), p. 17.
[571]   Ibid., pp. 20–21.
[572]   Richard Dawkins, 'A Reply to Poole', *Science & Christian Belief*, 7:1, No. 1 (1995), 45–50.

Teilhard's thought is a fine modern example of reflecting on the old philosophical problem of 'the one and the many', of seeing the individual human being as part of the whole of humanity, and of seeing humanity as part of the stream of life within an evolutionary world and cosmos.

When speaking about science, Teilhard called it the 'twin sister of mankind'.[573] He acknowledged the great advances which science had made and remarked that 'the march of humanity, as a prolongation of all other animate forms, develops indubitably in the direction of a conquest of matter put to the service of mind'. With man's knowledge of hormones and the discovery of genes, Teilhard believed that it was only a matter of time before man could control the mechanism of organic heredity and eventually produce a new wave of organisms, an 'artificially provoked neo-life':

> Of old, the forerunners of our chemists strove to find the philosopher's stone. Our ambition has grown since then. It is no longer to make gold but life; and in view of all that has happened in the last fifty years, who would dare to say that this is a mere mirage?[574]

While saluting those who have the courage to see so far ahead, Teilhard reminds one and all that:

> However far science pushes its discovery of the 'essential fire' and however capable it becomes some day of remodelling and perfecting the human element, it will always find itself in the end facing the same problem—how to give to each and every element its final value by grouping them in the unity of an organized whole.[575]

His basic ideas revolve around the relation of human beings to humankind, humankind in relation to life and life in relation to the universe. In many ways one can consider his thought as being very ecological, for he could not see the human being except as part of nature, as being an integral part of the natural environment.

Teilhard did not stop at the natural evolution of the universe. He believed that biological evolution will be followed by a social and cultural evolution of the human community. This cultural evolution would lead to the development of one world civilization consisting of rich ethnic, cultural and religious diversities. To him the future was a great task, because it was in man's power to decide what kind of future he wished to shape. Thus, he argued, man was living

---

[573]   De Chardin, *Phenomenon of Man,* p. 248.
[574]   Ibid., pp. 250–51.
[575]   Ibid., p. 250.

a very important historical moment because he was at a new threshold where the future can no longer be taken for granted but had to be planned with great responsibility. In a situation of cross-cultural encounter and growing global interdependence, Teilhard's thought on evolution as a converging process is worth reflecting upon. He considers evolution as ultimately convergent, that is to say, as moving eventually towards greater unity, or towards unity-in-diversity:

> Teilhard's vision of the world is charged, therefore, with a deeper undertone of optimism; and in this it contrasts sharply with the sombre and pessimistic ideas propounded in recent years by certain philosophers and other writers. His message is one of hope and confidence. We learn from him not of anguish and nausea but of love—love of life and love for the world: not of 'aloneness' but of union.[576]

The human genome, as potential humanity, elicits our feelings of awe and respect because of what it is and what it will become. It exhibits a uniqueness which is not chemical or physical—it is a uniqueness which cannot be so reduced, without falsifying truth. It is a uniqueness which expresses the existence of an experiencing being with its primal consciousness. The new being, on to becoming a university professor, an astronaut or movie star, moves into the womb wall and by its primal consciousness, begins to unfurl the beauty of its human form, by incredibly complex processes.

It is amazing how the cells of the blastula rearrange themselves, eventually resulting in the transformation of the blastula into the intricate folded form of the early embryo or gastrula. This consists of three basic germ cell layers: the ectoderm which gives rise to the skin and nervous system; the mesoderm which gives rise to muscle and skeletal tissue; and the endoderm which gives rise to the lining of the gut with all its associated glands. What all this means is that potentiality must be there from the very beginning, from conception. The cells have inbuilt within them the programme of what they are to become. The dynamic of the information content in living things is not and cannot be explained by physics and chemistry. It is only by logical fallacies that we suppose that we have explained life by mechanistic analysis. Partly to blame for these logical fallacies is the field of bioethics itself because, in recent years, it has reached moral positions based on mistaken science.[577] Today, when we live in a society where modern science tends to reject as meaningless and useless, questions that

---

[576]   Wildiers, *Teilhard de Chardin*, p. 107.

[577]   Dianne N. Irving, *Can Either Scientific Facts or 'Personhood' Be Mediated?* <http://www.lifei ssues.net/writers/irv_13persomediated.html> [accessed 19 October 2004]

cannot be answered by it, there is an urgent need for a metaphysical foundation that can restore the respect, dignity and liberty that is due to man.

Philosophical reflection on the human genome will lead to a better understanding of its transcendental nature that is beyond the competence of science. It is our contention that since the launch of the HGP and the race that ensued for the patenting of human genes, the major players in the biotechnology industry focussed their attention on the 'without' of the human genome and in so doing, overlooked its 'within'. This is the classical debate between those who believe that there is no metaphysical reality that underlies the human genome and the others who believe that it is by working through the metaphysical nature of the human genome that we will be able to comprehend its true essential nature. When Arvid Pardo proposed to make the resources of the deep seabed and ocean floor the common heritage of mankind, he was afraid that if his idea of international management of these resources did not become a reality, then most of these resources would end up in the hands of the few technologically advanced nations that had the capability to explore and exploit these resources. Pardo wanted to avoid this and his *point de force* was that these resources were part of the common heritage and therefore no country had the right to appropriate any part of this common heritage. As shown earlier in this study, when Pardo proposed the concept of common heritage of mankind, he was not suggesting a new moral political innovation but rather he was reiterating a universal and intertemporal moral principle that was derived from natural law. So in a sense, the resources of the deep seabed and ocean floor represented, to Arvid Pardo, a reality that transcended their immediate existence as collections of manganese and cobalt nodules among other minerals—the nodules were not just any nodules but nodules that were part of the common heritage of mankind! The purpose of our research is to show that the same reasoning can be applied to the human genome in the sense that it represents a reality that transcends its immediate existence as a collection of human genes in that embodies our very humanness that is a safeguard of both our individual and species-identity. It is our common heritage and at the same time it is *who we are*. But as a transcendental reality the human genome is also projected towards the future and as responsible stewards of the human genome that is our common heritage, we must respect the right of future generations to an unmanipulated human genome. As stewards of the human genome that is our common heritage, we have the right to use the human genome for and on behalf of all mankind but we do not have the right to own it—we certainly do not have the right to change it. For Habermas, any attempt to 'alter the essence of another human being' was a serious threat to the fundamental unity among men that comes from being 'grown' rather than 'made'.[578]

3.6   A Thought Experiment

Geneticists tell us that a fair amount of the DNA found in all organisms serves as some function that is as yet unknown. This DNA is normally referred to as Junk-DNA. Now, considering the fact that there is an enormous amount of this junk-DNA, could it not be the case that this sea of DNA is a form of latent information that is only meant to trigger activity within the human organism when environmental conditions are right? The DNA is only junk-DNA to us, with the current scientific knowledge at our disposal that is always temporary and incomplete. And so, could it be remotely possible that in the future, this junk-DNA, or more appropriately this limitless sea of genes, begins to mutate and forge into a transformed humanity the moment the biosphere reaches a critical level of evolutionary maturity. In this imaginary scenario, the possibilities are endless, considering the profundity of DNA and its limitless capacity to organize chemical and biological processes.

To Teilhard, this transformed humanity will 'detach itself from this planet and join the one true, irreversible essence of things, the Omega point'.[579] For Teilhard, the Omega point was Jesus Christ and exactly because it is Jesus Christ, his theory is unpalatable to most scientists!

3.7   Of Genomes and Souls

It is Aritstotle's metaphysics that can provide a solid foundation for our understanding of human nature and the human genome and for this reason we must embark on a work of retrieving the salient aspects of Aristotle's philosophy to represent them to the modern world in order to reaffirm the transcendent nature of our humanness and to stop us on the road to the dehumanization of man that is this century's most perilous threat to mankind.

---

[578]   Jurgen Habermas, *The Future of Human Nature* (Cambridge: Polity Press, 2003), p. 23.
[579]   De Chardin, *Vision of the Past*, pp. 52–57.

According to Aristotle, living things are substances that have an internally defining essence that informs and unifies their parts and properties.[580] Hence they constitute a unity that has qualities that do not stand outside of it.[581] It follows that a human being is the way he or she is because he or she possesses an internal essence that defines and orders his or her properties and is more than the external organization of his or her parts functioning in a given way. Its properties are deeply unified and related internally as part of the essential nature of humanness.

For Aristotle,[582] it is only possible for substances to possess an internal nature. The essential nature of substance informs their being and gives them the essential properties that are characteristic of their natural kind. All members of the same species express the same essential nature because it is this that directs the developmental process of the substance and establishes limits on the variations each substance may undergo and still exist. A human embryo functions in light of what it is and maintains its essence regardless of the degree to which its ultimate capacities are realized. While there may be variations among the individual members of a class of substances, such variance does not affect the essential nature of their being because it is the underlying essence of a thing and not its state of development at a given point that constitutes what it is.[583] The development and realization of its potential or its capacities are controlled by the substance's essential nature and so it does not become more of its kind but rather it matures according to its kind. The capacities for the human embryo to develop a brain, heart and lungs are already embedded within the human embryo prior to their realization. Whether or not the human embryo actually develops into a full-grown human adult depends on conditions such as the health of the mother carrying the embryo and the absence of potentially dangerous substances such as drugs and alcohol in the mother's blood stream. Hence, the embryo has capacities that are latent and will be expressed if conditions are right for their development. If the human embryo fails to develop, it is the fault of the conditions, not of the natural essence or nature.

---

[580] Sir David Ross, *Aristotle* (London: Routledge, 1996), p. 171.

[581] Aristotle, *The Metaphysics,* trans. by Hugh Lawson-Tancred (London: Penguin Books, 2004), pp. 248–49.

[582] Ibid., pp. 272–77.

[583] Scott B. Rae and Paul M. Cox, *Bioethics: A Christian Approach in a Pluralistic Age* (Michigan: William B. Eerdmans Publishing Company, 1999), pp. 159–60.

For Aristotle, substances maintain their ontological identity through change. A human organism is an ontological whole whose parts, properties and capacities are related internally.[584] A human being has a human identity of bodily organs and structures of consciousness, which presuppose the human essence of which the organs and structures are a part. For this reason, every human being exhibits behaviour that is specific to the human species, such as rational thought and the use of language, strongly suggesting an essential nature that is common to all members of the human species. From Aristotle-the-Biologist's point of view, before fertilization there are two natures, i.e., the nature of an ovum and the nature of a sperm. After fertilization there is a human [zygote] with one nature, i.e., the nature of a human being. Therefore, in fertilization there is a substantial change because the substances or natures of the ovum and the sperm have changed into the nature of a human being.[585] This is, in fact, known empirically by observing the number and the kinds of chromosomes present before and after fertilization, and by empirically observing the different characteristically specific actions and functions of the ovum, the sperm and the human zygote. Once fertilization has taken place and the new human being has formed, the nature of the human being does not change but only its human accidents change.

Modern Thomists have reinterpreted the notion of soul in genomic terms in order to make it compatible with the thesis that a person comes into being at fertilization when a zygote is formed from the fusion of two gametes with separate and distinct genomes.[586] The new diploid genome coincides with the emergence of a new organism and contains the genetic programme that will direct the development of that organism. Furthermore, the new genome remains stable throughout an individual's life and so is the biological precondition for both species-identity and personal-identity. Thus embryological development does not entail substantial change, but only accidental change. Once it is a human being it stays a human being and acts and functions biologically as a human being. The human zygote produces specifically human enzymes and proteins;

---

[584]   Aristotle, *Physics*, trans. by Robin Waterfield (Oxford: Oxford University Press, 1996), 2.1.192b, 8-32, pp. 33–34.

[585]   Ibid.,1.7.191a, 15–18, pp. 27–28; 2.3.194b, 23–35, p. 39.

[586]   Mauron, 'Is the Genome the Secular Equivalent of the Soul?', pp 831–32.

he or she forms specifically human tissues and organ systems and develops humanly and continuously from the stage of a single-cell human zygote embryo to the stage of a human adult.[587]

With regards to the human embryo, Aquinas asserts that 'just as the soul in an embryo is in act, but imperfectly, so also it operates, but imperfect operations',[588] where by the soul being 'in act', he refers to a soul being present in a human embryo as its first actuality. In saying that the soul being 'imperfectly in act', he is referring to the fact that a human embryo does not exhibit all the soul's powers as second actualities. Aquinas' conclusion is that a soul operates in a human embryo as its substantial form and in the actual exercise of at least vegetative and possibly also sensitive operations but it initially only performs 'imperfect operations' in that it does not fully exercise all its proper operations until later in the embryo's development.

In short, the biological facts demonstrate that at fertilization we have a real human being with a truly human nature. It is not that he or she will become a human being—he or she already is a human being. We know this empirically and this nature or capacity to act in a certain characteristic way is called philosophically, a nature or potency. Thus a human zygote or embryo is not a possible human being; he or she is already a human being. A human zygote, embryo or foetus does not have the potency to become a human being, but already possesses the nature or capacity to be at that moment a human being. It is this same nature that will direct the accidental development, i.e., the embryological development of his or her own self from the most immature to the most mature stage of a human being.[589]

According to Aristotle, all natural beings have an internal and immanent purposiveness inherent in their generation, structure and activities.[590] The organism, guided by its self-contained end or *entelechy*, develops, unfolds and informs itself from within in successive stages that tend towards and reach a limit which is none other than itself, the fully formed organism. The emergence of the differentiating parts of the whole is coordinated, each part being related always to every part but also, prospectively, to the mature form of itself and of the whole.

---

[587] Keith l. Moore, *The Developing Human: Clinically Oriented Embryology*, 3rd edn. (Philadelphia: WB Saunders Company, 1982), p. 14.

[588] Eberl, Jason T., *Thomistic Principles and Bioethics* (London: Routledge, 2006).

[589] Aristotle, 'On the Soul' in *The Complete Works of Aristotle*, ed. by Jonathan Barnes, 2 vols (Princetown: Princetown University Press, 1995) 2.4.415b, 8–14, p. 661.

[590] Aristotle, *Physics*, trans. by Robin Waterfield (Oxford: Oxford University Press, 1999), II.8.199b, 26–31, p. 53.

The adult that emerges from the process of self-development and growth is no mere outcome but a completion, an end, a whole. The internal essence directs the developmental process and establishes limits on the variations it may undergo.

While for Aquinas the change required for something to actualize an active or passive potentiality is brought about by its 'proper active principle', he did not believe that the human zygote actually possessed such a principle, which meant that it lacked the potential to develop the proper organs required for rational thought necessary for a human being to achieve its *entelechy*. But this lack of recognition on the part of Aquinas is due to the lack of awareness on his part of the way DNA functions in a zygote or early embryo to guide its natural development such that it comes to have the requisite organs. Aquinas mistakenly postulated a 'formative power' transmitted to the zygote and early embryo by the semen which then guides its development.[591] Our understanding of DNA puts this 'formative power' directly within the zygote or early embryo with the semen losing its role as 'carrier and guide' of the same 'formative power'.[592]

Traditionally, it was believed that the rational soul, responsible for organizing and directing embryological development, was not infused in the developing foetus before three months. But if this were so, how could one explain the specifically human organization of the embryo and the human foetus up to that point? Modern scientific embryology provides us with empirical evidence that certain specific human functions and activities, such as the production of human proteins, enzymes and so on, are also present from the very beginning. Hence, if this complex human structural organization exists from the very beginning then it follows, by necessity, that the soul is also present from the very beginning! For both Aristotle and Aquinas, the rational soul is not an entity separate from the vegetative and sensitive parts—the Thomistic-Aristotelain idea of soul comprises the total complexity of the human structure, incorporating both form and matter.[593] In other words, the totality of the human person is made up of both body and soul and together they constitute one homogeneous substance.[594]

---

[591]   Eberl, *Thomistic Principles and Bioethics*, p. 29.

[592]   Ibid.

[593]   Aristotle, 'On the Soul', 1.5.411b, 14-18, pp. 655–56; 1.5.411b, 24-28, p. 656.

[594]   St. Thomas Aquinas, *Summa Theologiae: The Trinity*, ed. / trans. by Timothy Sutton, 60 vols (London: Blackfriars, 1975), VI, pp. 41–47. (ST, 1a, q.29, a. 1).

It is the same DNA that is shared by all living organisms—all living organisms come to be as a result of numerous biochemical reactions coded for, specified, regulated, directed and ordered by the respective blueprints of the different organisms. It is the same DNA that, depending on the *in-form-ation* of the particular species, produces totally different organisms. Hence, although the genetic code and the machinery for its translation are, for the most part, uniform and universal, the ordered expression of genes and the overall organization of the genetic messages in each organism bear the unmistakable stamp of the species-specific form.

As mentioned earlier, every living being has its *entelechy* or self-contained end or purpose. So, the parts of an organism, such as the bone marrow and the heart, have their own specific functions which define their nature as parts—the bone marrow makes red blood cells while the heart pumps blood. Even at the biochemical level, every molecule has a specific function which defines its nature: haemoglobin is a protein that phosphylates glucose. There is also a co-relation between the complexity of the biochemical structure of the molecule and the complexity of its functional capabilities. DNA polymerase, for example, is a protein that copies the existing DNA molecules, faithfully reproducing the sequence of the bases so that the encoded messages are not scrambled when the cells multiply and divide. Enzymes that produce genetic novelty, mutations that have a specific function and even the production of apparently accidental variations are activities which, to some extent, elicit an organic or purposive activity. Hence, all the parts of an organism, both macroscopic and microscopic, have functional capabilities which contribute towards the proper functioning of the other parts and the proper functioning of the organism as a whole.

Living organisms are not only self-producing, self-organizing, self-maintaining, self-preserving and self-fulfilling but also self-healing. It is a power which enables living organisms to heal wounds and regain wholeness from within their very being. In higher animals, the immune system is able to reject any foreign bodies such as infectious agents or graft tissues in order to maintain their wholeness. They display a 'striving forward' that characterizes most of their activities.[595] Hence, a young bird will remain in its nest and continue to struggle to coordinate wing and tail motions before it ventures to fly, and for the same reasons but with a different purpose, a seedling sprouting beneath a large rock will bend and grow around the rock to reach the light. Again, for the same reasons but for a totally different purpose, the peacock will dance before the

---

[595]   Aristotle, *Physics*, 2.8. 198b 10-199a 15, pp. 50–51.

female in order to mate with her. These animal activities, albeit not being conscious or intended, demonstrate, without any shred of doubt, a directed, inwardly determined activity with a specific end and for a specific purpose.

The notion of a human being as a substance has great significance for the moral status of the human genome. Viewing human beings as substances that have continuity of personal identity through change suggests that from the moment of the fusion of the two human gametes, a new human embryo with a new genome commences a continuous process of growth and development which culminates in an adult human being.[596] It is important to note that there is no *break* in the process of development. This is a very significant fact which must, of necessity, underlie the moral status of the human genome. The conclusion that the human embryo is a person from the moment of conception onwards follows from the true premises that human beings are the result of a continuous growth process and that there is no morally relevant break in the process. The force of the argument clearly rests on the second premise, that there is no morally relevant break in the development from conception to adulthood. Since virtually everyone agrees that once a child is born, he or she is a full person with all the corresponding rights to life, one could state this premise more specifically as that there is no morally relevant break in the process between conception and birth.[597]

By placing all our hopes in our genes we are fuelling the expectation that the human genome will be the last word on human nature. But this expectation is an illusion which may lead to the dehumanization of the human condition that needs a fresh philosophical start that cannot be provided by genomics alone!

3.8   The Human Difference

Jurgen Habermas, in his book *The Future of Human Nature*, expresses a number of concerns which are shared by many people who are preoccupied with the dehumanization effect which bad science can have on future generations. Habermas warns his readers that in our regulation of genetic engineering we should be guided by the question of:

---

[596]   Germain G. Grisez, *Abortion: The Myths, the Realities and the Arguments* (New York: Corpus Books, 1970), p. 275.

[597]   Dianne N. Irving, *Philosophical and Scientific Analysis of the Nature of the Early Human Embryo*, <http://www.lifeissues.net/writers/irv/irv_36whatisbioethics12.html> [accessed on 23 November 2004]

...the meaning, for our own life prospects and for our self-understanding as moral beings, of the proposition that the genetic foundations of our existence should not be passed over.[598]

He writes in favour of the right to an unmanipulated genetic heritage and points out that as gene manipulation touches the core of our identity as human beings, it threatens our conceptions of law and morality which are built on the anthropological self-understanding of the species. In other words, if genetic manipulation is allowed to change the self-understanding of the species in such a way that our conceptions of law and morality are put into question, then the 'inalienable normative conceptions of societal integration' will also be affected'.[599]

Hans Jonas expresses the same concerns when he writes that the

...more ruthless the intrusion into the makeup of the human genome becomes, the more inextricably the clinical mode of treatment is assimilated to the biotechnological mode of intervention, blurring the intuitive distinction between the grown and the made, the subjective and the objective—with repercussions reaching as far as the self-reference of the person to her bodily existence.[600]

Symbolically the human genome stands for all that which makes us human. With the completion of the HGP, the human genome has become more susceptible to commodification and commercialization. With the UNESCO Declaration on the Human Genome and Human Rights of 1997, the world community took the first step towards realizing the project of managing the human genome and the biomedical inventions that may be derived from it, as a common heritage of mankind, as originally envisaged by Arvid Pardo. Our study considers it imperative that the world community assumes its responsibilities and obligations as a trustee on behalf of mankind and embarks on a journey that will only reach its end when the concept of common heritage of mankind, as applied to the human genome, is not merely a philosophical concept but an international legal norm with clear provisions applicable in all states that are members of the UN General Assembly.

The object of the next section of our study will be to examine, from a philosophical perspective, the biotechnology that is being employed by biotech companies to exploit the human genome. This will be followed with concrete politico-ethical proposals for the development of a humane and compassionate

---

[598] Habermas, *The Future of Human Nature*, 2005, pp. 22–23.
[599] Ibid., p. 26.
[600] Hans Jonas, *Lasst uns einen Menschen klonieren*, quoted in Habermas, *The Future of Human Nature*, 2005, p. 47.

health care system that would rather treat patients as persons rather than as androids. In order to achieve such a goal, we must have the courage to do the things that we have to do and refrain from doing the things that we should not do! In the words of Paul Ramsey, we must, Raise the ethical questions with a serious and not a frivolous conscience.

> A man of frivolous conscience announces that there are ethical quandaries ahead that we must urgently consider before the future catches up with us. By this he often means that we need to devise a new ethics that will provide the rationalization for doing in the future what men are bound to do because of new actions and interventions science will have made possible. In contrast a man of serious conscience means to say in raising urgent ethical questions that there may be some things that men should never do. The good things that men do can be made complete only by the things they refuse to do.[601]

---

[601]   Paul Ramsey, *Fabricated Man: The Ethics of Genetic Control* (New Haven: Yale University Press, 1970), pp. 122–23.

Chapter Four
Questioning the Nexus Between Biotechnology and the Human Genome

4.1 In the Shadow of Technology

The next section of our study will focus on the technology that is being employed in the field of human genomic research. Many are concerned that modern science, with its penchant for gaining mastery over nature, including the human genome, has transformed the way we relate with ourselves, with others and with the world around us. 'Man has Nature whacked' is a friend's comment that C.S. Lewis reports in his essay, *The Abolition of Man.*[602] But immersed as we are within a technological culture that provides us with new gadgets with each day that passes, we remain oblivious to the dangers that are inherent in the new technology that is at the same time 'whacking' Nature.

It was Heidegger who identified modern technology as the principal danger of our time. He saw modern technology's relation to nature as more of a 'challenging-forth' involving the harnessing of power and energy rather than a 'bringing-into-being' of machines and tools.[603] Other philosophers have shown similar concerns about modern technology and the threat it poses to humankind.[604] My particular interest lies in the threats to the human genome that are inherent in the field of biotechnology. The commercialization of the human genome is but one symptom of the instrumental stance that modern science has adopted in relation to the human genome with devastating consequences that touch the core of our humanness. As such the problem does not lie with technology itself or biotechnology for that matter, but rather with man's 'relation' to technology and biotechnology.

Habermas, for example, argues that while in order to develop technology we must be able to see ourselves as 'the authors of our own histories', i.e., as

---

[602] C.S. Lewis, *The Abolition of Man* (New York: HarperCollins Publishers, 2001), p. 53.
[603] Heidegger, 'The Question Concerning Technology', pp. 320–28.
[604] Notably among these philosophers who have tackled the question of technology we find Jurgen Habermas, Hans-Georg Gadamer and Hans Jonas who have all been trained in the philosophical thought of Martin Heidegger.

autonomous beings, the technology being developed today is undermining this very feature of our humanity.[605] Jacques Ellul, another philosopher who has written extensively on the subject, speaks of technology as an entire way of being that, driven by a rational impulse to order all aspects of our world toward efficiency and control, is set to achieve the highest efficiency at the least possible cost and trouble.[606] The problem with technology is that, in principle, it is beyond human control. Ellul argues that although we may appear to be choosing between a better and worse technology, this is only an illusion because in actual fact our choice would be made automatically in favour of that technique that is considered the most efficient by way of eliminating all hitherto non-technical aspects of life.[607] Martin Heidegger, whose essay *The Question Concerning Technology* is considered the first major philosophical work on the subject, argues on the same lines when he explains that our response to the various problems raised by technology cannot be solved by just making technology better because the problem lies in our orientation to technology:

> Thus we shall never experience our relationship to the essence of technology so long as we merely conceive and push forward the technological, put up with it, or evade it. Everywhere we remain unfree and chained to technology, whether we passionately affirm or deny it.[608]

The next section of our study will deal with the problems surrounding technology and biotechnology and the ways they can lead to a shrunken self-understanding of the species. These problems have a direct bearing on the process of making the human genome the common heritage of mankind. So the role of the philosopher in dealing with the essence of technology becomes that of a 'watchman' who must remain on the alert to promote the human person towards its full realization and to detect whatever may prove deleterious in achieving this goal.[609] This is particularly true of genetic technology that threatens to deny the human person the right to a genetic inheritance that is immune from artificial intervention. Several scientists have shown an interest in manipulating the hu-

---

[605]   Jurgen Habermas, *The Future of Human Nature* (Cambridge: Polity Press, 2005), pp. 23–29.

[606]   Jacques Ellul, *The Technological Society*, trans. by John Wilkinson (New York: Vintage Books, 1964), p. 21.

[607]   Ibid., p. 99.

[608]   Heidegger, 'The Question Concerning Technology', p. 311.

[609]   Gabriel Marcel, *Man Against Mass Society*, trans. by G.S. Fraser (Chicago: Gateway, 1952), pp. 103–32.

man genome and taking evolution in their own hands with unimaginable consequences for the self-understanding of the human species.[610] This may threaten
the foundations of law and morality together with the 'inalienable normative
foundations of societal integration'.[611] The philosopher's task is to watch over
the biotechnology debate so as not to allow the technological disposition to proceed to its self-augmenting limits but rather bring it under intellectual, spiritual,
moral and political rule.

4.2   Unconcealing the Concealed in Technology

The question of technology and the way it bears an influence on human life was
first raised by Martin Heidegger and all other major philosophers who have written on the same theme have by and large taken their main ideas from Heidegger.
For him, the issue is not technology in itself but rather, man's relation to technology.[612] This is the basis of Heidegger's concern with technology which is
always taken for granted as a given by the majority of contemporary philosophers and scientists. And this is also where the problem lies with the human
genome because if we do not deliberately choose to take a step backwards away
from biotechnology and by doing so, move from a subjective to an objective
stance towards it, then our reflection on the role of biotechnology in relation to
our human genome will be shrouded by a veil of ignorance that jeopardizes our
cognizance of the dangers that biotechnology poses to the human genome and
concomitantly, humankind.

The same philosophical concerns that spurred Heidegger to write about
technology prompted Arvid Pardo to propose to the international community
that the deep seabed be made the common heritage of mankind. Addressing the
Committee on the Peaceful Uses of the Seabed and the Ocean Floor on 23 March
1971, Pardo had said:

> Man has now acquired the capability, not, of course to make the oceans disappear, but to
> impair their ability to sustain life and to serve his activities usefully. No nation or state is likely
> to destroy an environment vital to our existence deliberately, since such an act would serve
> no useful purpose, but the modern world is caught in what seems a fatal course of events.
> Rapid and ever more widespread industrialization and urbanization, accompanied by increas-
> ingly intense activities in ocean space, make it extremely difficult to arrest what could become,

---

[610]   Habermas, *The Future of Human Nature*, 2005, p. 42.
[611]   Ibid., p. 26.
[612]   Heidegger, 'The Question Concerning Technology', p. 311.

in a generation or two, the irresponsible contamination of the greater part of the world's water resources.[613]

It was in his probing of the relation between the technological disposition and the self-identity of the human species that Arvid Pardo has been singled out as a powerful figure in intellectual history. To many he is a path breaker who introduced, in the international political arena, a completely new form of international management of the world's deep seabed resources. Pardo's concept of common heritage of mankind has also been applied to outer space, the moon and Antarctica, as explained earlier in our study.

In proposing to make the deep seabed the common heritage of mankind, Pardo had said:

The dark oceans were the womb of life: from the protecting oceans life emerged. We still bear in our bodies—in our blood, in the salty bitterness of our tears—the marks of this remote past. Retracing the past, man, the present dominator of the emerged earth, is now returning to the ocean depths. His penetration of the deep could mark the beginning of the end for man, and indeed for life as we know it on this earth.[614]

One can only surmise, after reading these words coming from the lips of Arvid Pardo, that, like Heidegger before, Pardo was very much concerned that, to use Heidegger's interpretation of man as 'standing reserve', modern technology would soon transform people from 'free agents' to 'natural resources' that would then be exploited as 'standing reserve'.[615] There were two things that Pardo wanted to prevent and these were: (i) the unilateral exploitation of the natural resources of the planet by the industrialized nations that alone had the technology to do so, to the detriment of less industrialized nations who, legitimately, wanted their own share of these natural resources, and (ii) the dehumanization of mankind that he was sure would inevitably follow if the technological disposition was allowed to proceed, unchecked. For these reasons, Pardo wanted the natural resources of the deep seabed to be exploited within the context of a New International Economic Order by an international authority for and on behalf of all mankind.[616]

---

[613]   Pardo, *The Common Heritage of Mankind*, pp. 189–90.

[614]   Ibid., p. 2.

[615]   Heidegger, 'The Question Concerning Technology', pp. 321–22.

[616]   Address by Arvid Pardo to the 22nd Session of the General Assembly of the United Nations (1967), Official Records of the General Assembly, Twenty-Second Session, Agenda Item 92, Document A/6695.

In proposing to make the human genome the common heritage of mankind, the role of the philosopher as watchman becomes more demanding when we are talking about our identity as human beings. One need only to recall Article One of the Universal Declaration on the Human Genome and Human Rights which states that:

> The human genome underlies the fundamental unity of all members of the human family, as well as the recognition of their inherent dignity and diversity. In a symbolic sense, it is the heritage of humanity.[617]

Two were the senses that the drafters had in mind when they used the term 'genome' in the declaration, namely that of 'full set of genes of the individual' and the 'entire range of genes which constitute the human race'. By employing the term 'genome' in a metonymic sense, the drafters incorporated the twin meanings of the human genome, which can be surmised as the individual human genome that is representative of the collective human genome of the whole species. The vulnerability of human nature to man's technological intervention cannot be underestimated. The same can be said for biotechnological interventions on the human genome.

4.3   Transforming Technology

The first assertion that Heidegger makes with regards to the nature of technology concerns its mode of revealing. According to him, technology presents itself as a 'challenging forth' that transforms nature into a quantifiable resource or energy reserve that can be stored and disposed of independently of its originating context. So, when the River Rhine becomes an energy resource for hydroelectric turbines to generate electric energy, it becomes no different from coal mines or nuclear power plants that also produce electric energy. As a 'standing reserve', the generation of hydroelectric energy ceases to be dependent on natural factors such as the flow of the river.[618] This relation of technology towards nature has little to do with the artistic stance that expresses itself as a 'bringing forth' with the windmill seen as a source of natural energy when air flows through its sails and makes them move. Here, the generation of natural energy remains dependent on natural factors, namely the air flowing through the sails and making them

---

[617]   Universal Declaration on the Human Genome and Human Rights, adopted by the General Conference of UNESCO at its 29th Session on 11 November 1997, Article 1.

[618]   Heidegger, 'The Question Concerning Technology', p. 321.

move.[619] Likewise the human genome is being 'challenged-forth' into being a 'DNA repository' that, as 'standing reserve', is waiting to be exploited as a human resource. Again, this form of 'challenging-forth' has little to do with the 'bringing-forth' of the human genome as a revealing of its essential nature as the embodiment of our humanness. This is the kind of threat that biotechnology poses to the human genome when it obfuscates its true nature that has nothing to do with it being a 'DNA repository'.

It was in his *Contributions to Philosophy*,[620] which he wrote between 1936 and 1938, that Heidegger first reflected at length on the issue of technology. Here he speaks of the technological approach to the world as 'machination' intending to mean the same mode of being of technology in relation to the world that he elucidates in his *The Question Concerning Technology* of 1953. By 'machination' Heidegger refers to the way technology imposes upon the natural world, including human beings, to be a 'standing reserve' or, as Richard Polt put it rather bluntly, 'as one big gas station'.[621]

In asserting that the essence of technology has nothing to do with anything technological, Heidegger is able to move the discussion of technology from the field of technological experts to the field of philosophy where he is the expert. He is then able to retrieve the rich sources of the essence of technology which he demonstrates as being antecedent to the different technologies, including biotechnologies that have mushroomed since the eighteenth and nineteenth centuries.

Heidegger sets about to question the role of technology in our lives because he believes that we can only establish a free relationship with it if we are able to see it for what it is. In a word, we need to uncover the true essence of technology if we wish to relate to it as free agents. Heidegger's assertion that technology is relentlessly overtaking us should not come to us as a surprise when we look at the way things have evolved in the world of production with most natural things looked upon as 'natural resources', including human beings that have become *human resources* and the human genome that has become a *human databank*. With digital technology, the accessibility and manipulation of data have increased to an extent that was never imagined possible up to a few years ago.

---

[619]   Ibid., p. 320.
[620]   Martin Heidegger, *Contributions to Philosophy (From Enowning)*, trans. by Parvis Emad Emad and Kenneth Maly (Bloomington, Indiana: Indiana University Press, 1999), pp. 88–90.
[621]   Richard Polt, *Heidegger* (London: Routledge, 2003), p. 171.

Consider for example the digital archive of no less than 23 CD ROMS of three-dimensional images created by the Visible Human Project[622] from two human cadavers using the latest CT and MRI technology and the creation of Gen-Bank[623] with around 85,759,586,764 bases in 82,853,685 sequence records as of January 2008!

Technology is normally understood as a means to an end and the technological enterprise is driven by the desire to master technology by manipulating it to our advantage.[624] Every attempt to bring man into the right relation to technology is conditioned by the instrumental stance of technology in relation to man. Heidegger does not deny that technology is a means to an end but he goes far beyond the predominantly instrumental definition of technology. What is at stake for Heidegger is how we, as *Dasein*, can establish a free relationship with technology. And this relationship will only be truly free if it is able to open our human existence to the essence of what technology is. However, for Heidegger, in order to achieve this, the inadequacy of the instrumental definition of technology to demonstrate technology's true essence must be revealed. Charles Taylor argues along the same lines when he explains that the debased and mechanistic world view of today, brought about by an urbanized technological society, has obscured the spiritual reality behind nature and 'uncorrupted human feeling'. He also believes that the epiphany that will 'unshackle' us from the 'clasp' of technology must take into serious consideration the penchant of modern science, since the second half of the nineteenth century, to englobe within its grasp the life sciences as well.[625] The same must be said about the kind of human genomic research that is very often conducted according to criteria dictated solely

---

[622]   Visible Human Project – Begun in 1995 the US National Library of Medicine and the US National Institutes of Health created a digital archive of three-dimensional images of the human body from two donated corpses, an executed prisoner and a Maryland housewife. After the bodies were scanned using MRI technology, they were cryogenically frozen to -85 degrees Celsius in blue gelatin before being cut into four sections, each of which was CT and MRI scanned. These four sections were then planed at 1 millimeter intervals using a highly sophisticated piece of equipment called a cryomacrotome, to be CT scanned once again.

[623]   GenBank – It is the genetic sequence database of the US National Institutes of Health comprising all publicly available DNA sequences. It is part of the International Nucleotide Sequence Database Collaboration together with the DNA DataBank of Japan and the European Molecular Biology Laboratory. The three organizations exchange data on a daily basis.

[624]   Heidegger, 'The Question Concerning Technology', p. 313.

[625]   Charles Taylor, *Sources of the Self: The Making of the Modern Identity* (Cambridge: Cambridge University Press, 2006), pp. 456–57.

by economic considerations. This has resulted, to cite one example, in a total lack of private investment in the research and development of drugs for tropical diseases because this is not considered to be a profitable market—between 1975 and 1996, less than 1% of 1223 drugs sold worldwide were intended for tropical diseases![626]

For Heidegger, only an accurate analysis of the way the instrumental definition of technology employs the functional terms of 'means' and 'ends' will unmask the obstacles that obscure the path that will lead to an existential change from a subjectivist to an objectivist stance to the essence of technology where technology will be experienced within its own boundary conditions.[627]

Heidegger reminds us that 'a means is that whereby something is effected and thus attained'.[628] And, 'whatever has an effect as its consequence is called a cause'.[629] But, according to Heidegger, 'not only that by which something is effected is a cause' because even 'the end that determines the kind of means to be used may also be considered a cause'.[630] At this point Heidegger returns to the sources of causality by employing Aristotle's doctrine of the four causes to reveal the true nature of technology. However, he goes further because his delving into the question of technology makes him doubt a number of things, such as whether the causes may be five or more rather than four or whether it is correct to presuppose that 'the causal character of the four causes is so unifiedly determined that they belong together?'[631]

Heidegger questions the presupposition that cause can be explained as 'that which brings something about' in the sense of 'effecting' because even though in the Aristotelian doctrine of causality, the *causa efficiens* is understood as 'that which brings it about that something turns out as result in such and such a way', this meaning of the term *causa* can be traced to a period in Greek thought that comes after Aristotle. The meaning of the Greek word *aiton* that Aristotle uses, which comes from an earlier period of Greek thought, carries the sense of 'that

---

[626]   Christian Lenk, Nils Hoppe and Roberto Andorno, *Ethics and Law of Intellectual Property: Current Problems in Politics, Science and Technology* (Aldershot: Ashgate Publishing Company, 2007), pp. 178–79.

[627]   Heidegger, 'The Question Concerning Technology', pp. 313–15.

[628]   Ibid., p. 313.

[629]   Ibid.

[630]   Ibid.

[631]   Ibid., p. 314.

to which something is indebted'.[632] So the four causes are the ways of 'being responsible for something else'.[633] And, in order to truly understand causality, we must uncover the true meaning that Aristotle intended by the notion of 'that which is responsible for something else'.[634]

Using the example of a silver chalice, Heidegger remarks that silver is 'co-responsible' for the chalice as it is the material or *hyle* from which the chalice is made.[635] But the 'indebtedness' of the chalice towards the silver goes beyond the material aspect of *hyle* to the form or *eidos* of chaliceness into which the silver is shaped. For Heidegger, both the silver as *hyle* or material and the *eidos* or form are 'co-responsible' for the chalice being a chalice.[636]

Telos is the third element that is co-responsible for the chalice together with *hyle* and *eidos* and it constitutes the defining boundaries of consecration and bestowal that give significance to the chalice prior to its actual production.[637] Finally the fourth participant in responsibility is the silversmith who, after careful consideration, brings the chalice into existence. Still, for Heidegger, even though the silversmith is responsible for bringing the chalice into existence, this has nothing to do with the fact that the silversmith is the actual chalice maker or *causa efficiens*—he does not see the silversmith as merely 'that which brings about' the chalice in the sense of 'effecting'. For Heidegger, the silversmith, after careful consideration, gathers together the three participants in responsibility mentioned before and 'brings forward into appearance' the chalice.[638]

The four ways of being responsible for the chalice 'bring-forth' the chalice out of concealment into unconcealment.[639] So the four *causes* are re-defined by Heidegger as four 'ways of being responsible' that 'assist' the potential chalice in the silver (*hyle*), in the idea of chaliceness (*eidos*), in the idea of consecration and bestowal (*telos*) and in making its appearance (*legein*).[640] At this point Heidegger postulates that technology is a kind of *poesis* or 'bringing forth' that

---

632 Heidegger, 'The Question Concerning Technology', p. 314.
633 Ibid.
634 O'Brien, '*Commentary on Heidegger's "The Question Concerning Technology"*', in *IWM Junior Visiting Fellows' Conferences*, Vol. XVI/I, 2004, pp. 1–38.
635 Heidegger, 'The Question Concerning Technology', p. 315.
636 Ibid.
637 Ibid.
638 For Heidegger, 'to consider carefully' is in Greek, *legein,* which is rooted in *apophainesthai* which means 'to bring forward'.
639 Heidegger, 'The Question Concerning Technology', pp. 317–18.
640 Ibid., p. 318.

'reveals something that has been concealed'. What is revealed from concealment for Heidegger is 'the realm of truth' that constitutes the 'essence of technology'.[641] This mode of revealing is naturally very different from the instrumental definition of technology as a way of getting things done.

So far Heidegger has made us return to the more fundamental ancient Greek meanings of terms commonly used in technological discourse. Although it cannot be denied that Heidegger is passionate about philosophical argumentation that is based upon etymology, one cannot help but admire his questioning concerning technology that has as its point of departure the Aristotelian paradigmatic account of causality that has shaped all future inquiries into technology.

The next stage of Heidegger's inquiry into the question of technology is focussed on the etymological origin of the term 'technology'. It in fact stems from the Greek word *technikon* which is related to the word *techne* that in Greek thought refers to both the activities and skills of the craftsman and the intellectual arts and the fine arts.[642] So at this point, *techne* may be considered a 'bringing-forth' or *poesis*. But, as Heidegger remarks, the word *techne* was, in Greek thought from Plato onwards, linked to the word *episteme* that has the sense of 'knowing'. From this connection between *techne* and *episteme*, Heidegger postulates that both words can be used for knowing in the widest sense:

> Thus what is decisive in *techne* does not at all lie in making and manipulating, nor in the using of means, but rather in the revealing mentioned before. It is as revealing, and not as manufacturing, that *techne* is a bringing-forth.[643]

So the essence of technology lies in 'revealing' and not in the actual making and manipulation of means towards ends. The silversmith, through *techne*, sets out to plan and bring to completion a project whereby he reveals that which as yet has not brought itself forth, by forging a chalice through the act of bringing together its matter and form, within the boundary definition of chaliceness.

In distinguishing between the essence of technology and the technological, Heidegger moves away from a predominantly mechanistic and reductionist un-

---

[641]   Heidegger arrives at this conclusion from the Roman translation *veritas* of the Greek word for revealing, *aletheia*. Hence the connection between 'revealing' and 'realm of truth'. The *aletheia* of technology is the space where revealing and unconcealment come together and truth happens!

[642]   Heidegger, 'The Question Concerning Technology', p. 318.

[643]   Ibid., p. 319.

derstanding of technology that has become so ingrained in modern society's collective imagination. Heidegger rejected the values of the city and technology and chose to spend as much time as possible in his cabin in the old town of Messkirch, near the Black Forest as he felt that he was more of a farmer than a city man.[644] Still he did not consider the technological as something evil or as something that we can do without.[645] But the point he makes is that we must respect the act of 'bringing forth' that is only made possible when man uses his intellect 'to bring X out of concealment into unconcealment'. In *The Thing* Heidegger comments on the making of a jug:

> The jug is not a vessel because it was made; rather, the jug had to be made because it is this holding vessel. The making...lets the jug come into its own. But that which in the jug's nature is its own is never brought about by its making.[646]

So X could be a 'jug' or it could be the human genome that the modern scientist, through *techne*, 'brings forth' on behalf and for the benefit of all mankind as a common heritage of mankind. The human genome, like the 'jug', 'comes into its own' and the nature of the human genome is not *made* by the scientist as the nature of the jug is not *made* by the artisan.

But X can also be made reducible to the technological as when the 'jug' is reduced to a mere utensil for containing liquids and the human genome is reduced to being a mere natural resource when, controlled and mastered by modern science, it is made subject to exploitation and manipulation in the interests of modern man who is blind to the dangers that are inherent in biotechnology as in all modern technology. Many are concerned that researchers and politicians in the UK have shown themselves to be so blind when the Human Fertilization and Embryology Authority (HFEA) decided in 2007 that there is no fundamental

---

[644] George Pattison, *The Later Heidegger* (London: Routledge, 2000), pp. 38–39.

[645] In Heidegger's infamous 'Memorial Address' he spoke of the arrangements, devices and machinery as being to a greater or less extent indispensable and claimed that it would be foolish to attack technology blindly and short sighted to consider it as the work of the devil. Reference to this address is made in 'Essays in Philosophy', by Ronald Godzinski Jr., in Vol. 6, No. 1, January 2005.

[646] Martin Heidegger, 'The Thing', in *Poetry, Language, Thought*, trans. by A. Hofstader (New York: Harper and Row, 1971), pp. 165–82.

reason to prevent cytoplasmic hybrid research.[647] Already in China there is reason to believe that researchers have been injecting rabbit eggs with human
DNA.[648] The whole question of chimeras and hybrids is very unsettling to those
who, like Jurgen Habermas, believe that humankind has the right to an unmanipulated genome. This is one of the reasons why it is imperative that every
effort is made to enact international and national legislation to establish the necessary regulation to protect the human genome from the mavericks of modern
science who act in ignorance of the fact that they themselves are cogs in the
wheels of the technological machine that they foolhardily think they have under
full control.[649] Tampering with the human genome is not an option considering
the catastrophic consequences that can result if things do not go exactly as
planned. When the prospect of cloning was first presented to the public in an
article published in 1966, Joshua Lederberg, a Nobel laureate geneticist, wrote:

> Then we must perform the algeny on gamete or zygote but in so doing we face the difficulty
> of testing the consequences of the intervention! If the purpose is a better human being, by any
> standard, we would face the same hazards generation after generation. The premise of this
> argument is that the inherent complexity of the system precludes any merely prospective ex-
> periment in algeny. It is bound to fail a large part of the time and possibly with disastrous
> consequences if we slip even a single nucleotide.[650]

In the same article, Lederberg argued that cloning could overcome the unpredictable variety which was common to natural reproduction and so could enable
prospective parents to produce progeny with enhanced genetic qualities such as
superior intelligence, memory or athletic ability. But in this scenario, the modern
scientist is not, through *techne*, 'bringing forth' what lies concealed in our human genome but rather he is subjecting the human genome to biotechnological
techniques to transform procreation into manufacture at the cost of denying human existence of such fundamental notions as identity, individuality, sexuality,

---

[647]   Michael Hopkin, 'Britain Gets Hybrid Embryo Go-Ahead', *Nature News* (5 September
2007/doi:10.1038/news070903-12). <http://www.nature.com/news/2007/070903/full/news07
0903-12.html> [accessed 20 January 2008]

[648]   Eric Cohen, *In the Shadow of Progress: Being Human in the Age of Technology* (New York:
Encounter Books, 2008), p. 28.

[649]   Hilde M. Zitzelsberger, 'Concerning Technology: Thinking with Heidegger', *Nursing Philosophy*, 5:3 (2004), pp. 242–50.

[650]   J. Ledeberg, 'Experimental Genetics and Human Evolution', *The American Naturalist*,
100:915 (1966), 519–31 (p. 526).

body and soul and lineage and kinship![651] It is unfortunate that when analytic philosophy took over the field of bioethics, many philosophers collectively abandoned their understanding and voices and contented themselves with merely abstractly analyzing new biotechnological developments as they emerged and allowing molecular biologists and biochemists to work outside the constraints of an ethics of medical practice.[652] Heidegger cannot be counted as being one of these philosophers because with his *The Question Concerning Technology* he succeeded in putting the technology question on the philosophical agenda of several philosophers who did not originate from the analytical school and who with their probing into the true nature of modern technology challenged the claims of modern science that there is no place for metaphysical explanations in the postmodern world.

It is to the question of modern technology that Heidegger now turns his attention. Before proceeding, however, it is to be noted that it is precisely in the area of biotechnology that the impotence of science to understand the truth about the human genome becomes readily apparent.

At the very start of his questioning into the nature of modern technology, Heidegger acknowledges that, on the one hand, it is different from the traditional technology that made the silver chalice or for that matter the techniques of the handicraftsman of classical times and, on the other hand, he asserts that in the final analysis, both forms of technology, the new and the old, are a form of re-vealing.[653] He then poses the question of whether modern technology is derived from modern physics or the other way round but he contends that irrespective of which position is correct, the crux of the matter lies in modern technology's orientation to the world.[654] And even though modern technology, like its traditional counterpart, is a mode of revealing, still it does not constitute a 'bringing-forth' or *poesis* where revealing and unconcealment come together and *aletheia*, truth happens.[655] Rather the revealing in modern technology is a 'challenging forth' that puts unreasonable demands on nature to supply energy that can be extracted and stored:

---

[651]   Kass, *Life, Liberty and the Defence of Dignity*, pp. 142–43.

[652]   Ramsey, *Fabricated Man*, pp. 104–05.

[653]   W.P.S. Dias, 'Heidegger's Relevance for Engineering: Questioning Technology', *Science and Engineering Ethics*, 9:3 (2003), 389–96.

[654]   Heidegger, 'The Question Concerning Technology', p. 320.

[655]   Ibid., p. 319.

The earth now reveals itself as a coal mining district, the soil as a mineral deposit. The field that the peasant formerly cultivated and set in order appears differently than it did when to set in order still meant to take care and maintain. The work of the peasant does not challenge the soil of the field. In sowing grain it places seed in the keeping of the forces of growth and watches over its increase. But meanwhile even the cultivation of the field has come under the grip of another kind of setting-in-order, which sets upon nature. It sets upon it in the sense of challenging it. Agriculture is now the mechanized food industry.[656]

The energy concealed in nature is unlocked to be transformed into an energy store. Technology is primarily concerned with the harnessing of power and energy, be it thermal, hydroelectric, chemical, solar or atomic.[657] And so it would seem that everywhere and everything is a 'standing reserve' as for example the airliner standing on the runway is not a mere 'object' but rather a 'standing reserve' in as much it is ordered, by the spirit of instrumental reason, to provide transportation.[658] Man is obviously the agent behind this challenging setting upon that demands of nature to be a 'standing reserve'. But he himself is 'challenged forth' as for example the forester, knowingly or not, must fell so many trees per week as demanded by the timber industry that is in turn 'challenged forth' by the demands of the cellulose industry which in turn is 'challenged forth' by the need for paper that is 'challenged forth' by the paper and magazine industry.[659] In a nutshell, technology's instrumental orientation to the world not only transforms the world into 'standing reserve' but also humanity. The same instrumental reasoning is behind the patenting system that is conducive to the creation of the *tragedy of the anti-commons* in biomedical research. A typical anti-commons is created when in order to claim an effective right to develop certain products such as therapeutic proteins or genetic diagnostic tests, a pharmaceutical company must pay costly transaction fees to many different owners of multiple patents on separate isolated gene fragments. The problem lies with allowing patents on newly identified DNA sequences, including the gene fragments in question before one can actually identify a corresponding gene, protein, biological function or potential commercial product.[660] These considerations put into question the *modus operandi* of the biotechnology industry that appears to be guided more by economic gain rather than by concerns of public health. A

---

[656]   Ibid., p. 320.
[657]   Kass, *Life, Liberty and the Defence of Dignity*, p. 32.
[658]   Heidegger, 'The Question Concerning Technology', p. 322.
[659]   Ibid., p. 323.
[660]   Heller and Eisenberg, 'Can Patents Deter Innovation', pp. 698–701.

case in point is the substance *eflornithine* that is an effective drug against sleeping sickness which threatens 60 million people each year. While *eflornithine* is not produced as a drug against sleeping sickness because of lack of profitability, the same substance is marketed in the form of a cream for the removal of facial hair by Bristol-Myers Squib, in co-operation with Gillette, as it is estimated that no less than 20 million women in the US remove their facial hair every week.[661]

For Hans Jonas, man himself has been added to the objects of technology. And in our contemporary culture, the human genome has suffered the same fate and, like man, has been added to the objects of technology, or more specifically, biotechnology. It follows, for Jonas that knowledge has become a prime duty and it should be commensurate with the causal scale of our action. We must be aware of how the technological/biotechnological modes of being put human nature, including the human genome, in a position of instrumental subjugation to them. But again, as the kind of knowledge that man seeks to acquire is only of a predictive nature which very often falls short of technical knowledge, the recognition of ignorance must constitute a fundamental consideration in our ethical thinking about the consequences that may result from technological and biotechnological innovation.[662]

Still according to Heidegger, although humanity is, so to speak, that which drives technology forward, it can never become mere raw material.[663] On the other hand, nature and nature's mode of revealing can never fall completely under human control, for even though we may and should control how we orient ourselves to natural resources such as coal or soil, we have no control over the formation of coal deposits and the accumulation of nitrogen in the soil.

> Since man drives technology forward, he takes part in ordering as a way of revealing. But the unconcealment itself, within which ordering unfolds, is never a human handiwork, any more than is the realm man traverses every time he as a subject relates to an object.[664]

The unconcealment of the unconcealed is not in the hands of man because he himself has been claimed by a mode of revealing that challenges him to see the world as a 'standing reserve'. Hans Jonas argues along the same lines when he

---

[661] Sterckx, 'Lack of Access to Essential Drugs', pp. 175–97.
[662] Jonas, *Philosophical Essays*, pp. 9–10.
[663] Heidegger, 'The Question Concerning Technology', p. 323.
[664] Ibid., pp. 323–24.

observes that with modern technology, developments set in motion by techno-logical acts with short-term goals tend to gather their own momentum to become not only irreversible but forward pushing to the point of overtaking the wishes and plans of the initiators. Jonas puts it succinctly when he says that, 'we are free at the first step but slaves at the second and all further ones'.[665] So one can-not really consider modern technology, as a revealing that challenges forth, the work of man because he essentially finds himself everywhere already brought into unconcealment to which he merely responds. Even still, man is never trans-formed into mere 'standing-reserve'.[666] This point is illustrated by Heidegger himself who instead of building his Black Forest farmhouse in the midst of a clearing in the forest requiring the cutting downs of trees and the levelling of the land, he contented himself with building the farmhouse *into* the hillside, allow-ing the natural landscape to protect it from the elements and provide the neces-sary conditions for living as a farmer.[667]

4.4   Technological Stewardship

Heidegger uses the term 'enframing' to describe the orientation humanity adopts in relation to the world. It has nothing to do with the technological domain of machines and other activities associated with modern modes of production. However, this does not spare technology from being itself conditioned by the process of 'enframing' that precedes it and challenges it to respond to its de-mands:

> Enframing means the gathering together of that setting-upon which rests upon man, i.e., chal-lenges him forth, to reveal the real, in the mode of ordering, as standing-reserve. Enframing means that way of revealing which holds sway in the essence of modern technology and which in itself is nothing technological. On the other hand, all those things that are so familiar to us and are standard parts of an assembly, such as rods, pistons and chassis, belong to the techno-logical. The assembly itself, however, together with the aforementioned stockparts, falls within the sphere of technological activity; and this activity always merely responds to the challenge of enframing, but it never comprises enframing itself or brings it about.[668]

So Heidegger's suggestion that modern technology has actually preceded and helped shape modern physics comes as no surprise, considering the human drive

[665]   Jonas, *The Imperative of Responsibility*,p. 32.
[666]   Heidegger, 'The Question Concerning Technology', p. 323.
[667]   Martin Heidegger, 'Building Dwelling Thinking' in *Basic Writings* (London: Routledge, 2007), pp. 343–63.
[668]   Heidegger, 'The Question Concerning Technology', p. 329.

behind the technological enterprise, to obtain a quantifiable and controllable knowledge of the world. He comes to this conclusion from an analysis of the word 'history' derived from the word *schicken* that means 'to send'. It was the human desire to build a comprehensive knowledge of the natural world that 'sent' humanity on the way to an orientation that viewed the world primarily as 'standing-reserve'. This eventually culminated in modern technology that overshadowed the primal relationship of the physical world to humanity on its own terms.[669]

Still, for Heidegger, the earlier relationship between the physical world and humanity has survived because despite the influence of modern technology on man's orientation to the world, humanity has continued to experience the physical world 'as the world reveals itself', notwithstanding the general tendency to experience it 'filtered' through the cage of technology. In other words, albeit 'enframing' puts man in a determined orientation to the world that is seen primarily as 'standing-reserve', man, by choice, remains free to allow the physical world to reveal itself to him on its own terms.

> It is precisely in enframing, which threatens to sweep man away into ordering as the ostensibly sole way of revealing, and so thrusts man into the danger of the surrender of his free essence— it is precisely in this extreme danger that the innermost indestructible belongingness of man within granting may come to light, provided that we, for our part, begin to pay heed to the essence of technology.[670]

Hence for Heidegger, it always remains possible for man to enter into a free relationship with technology as long as man's response to the act of revealing of the physical world to humanity remains one of contemplation. But what does man contemplate before the act of revealing of the physical world to him? It is none other than the Truth of Being or *Dasein*, over which, Heidegger believes, humanity was granted responsible stewardship:

> *Physis* also, the arising of something from out of itself, is a bringing-forth, *poiesis*. *Physis* is indeed *poiesis* in the highest sense. For what presences by means of *physis* has the bursting open belonging to bringing-forth, e.g., the bursting of a blossom into bloom, in itself (*en heautoi*).[671]

So for Heidegger, technology is not simply a means to an end but rather a way of revealing the world of Being and for this reason the essence of technology is

---

[669] Ibid.
[670] Ibid., p. 337.
[671] Ibid., p. 317.

the realm of Truth. Firmly believing that mankind has been granted the special role of 'Shepherds of Being', Heidegger insists that although the revealing at work within the essential realm of 'enframing' does not depend 'decisively' on man, still it has to happen 'exclusively' through him.[672] The problem is that man has been called to assume this responsible stewardship of Being after he himself has been 'challenged forth' by 'enframing' and logically this implies that man's relationship to the essence of technology 'always comes too late!' It follows that our call to act as 'Shepherds of Being' arises within the essential realm of 'enframing' and not outside of it. But this poses more of a challenge to Heidegger than a problem which he explains with the help of the poet, Frierich Holderlin:

But where danger is, grows
The saving power also.[673]

So, for Heidegger, the key to establishing a free relationship to technology lies within the essential realm of 'enframing' itself. But in order to arrive at this free relationship with technology, we must 'attune ourselves to the manner in which we are determined in advance by 'enframing'.[674]

Before proceeding with Heidegger's philosophical analysis of questions related to technology, it must be noted that Heidegger's thinking on the relation between the physical world and humanity can be directly applied to humanity's relation to the human genome. So, even though 'enframing' conditions man in the way he perceives the human genome which is seen primarily as a 'standing-reserve' or 'DNA repository' that is waiting to be exploited, still, we are free to allow the human genome to 'reveal' itself to us on its own terms. What is important for Heidegger is that our response to the act of revealing of, in our case, the human genome remains one of contemplation. And in so doing, we will be contemplating nothing less than the essential being of the human genome, or to put it more succinctly, its metaphysical nature. At this stage the role of the philosopher becomes one of 'Safekeeper of the Human Genome' in as much as he is the 'Safekeeper of the Truth of Being or *Dasein*'.[675] The unique relation between mankind and the human genome, as formulated by Heidegger in the wider

---

[672]   Mahon O'Brien, 'Commentary on Heidegger's "The Question Concerning Technology"', in *IWM Junior Visiting Fellows' Conferences*, Vol. XVI/I, 2004, p. 25.

[673]   Fiedrich Holderin, *Patmos in Poems and Fragments*, quoted in Heidegger, 'The Question Concerning Technology', p. 333.

[674]   O'Brien, 'Commentary on Heidegger's "The Question Concerning Technology"', p. 30.

[675]   Heidegger, 'The Question Concerning Technology', p. 339.

context of the relation of mankind with the physical world or *Dasein*, provides the ontological basis for mankind's role of responsible stewardship of the human genome. So, even though mankind is conditioned in its relation to the human genome as a result of the patenting system that has led to its commercialization, still mankind is free to rediscover a new orientation to the human genome if its approach to it remains one of contemplation rather than domination. Making the human genome the common heritage of mankind as originally envisaged by Arvid Pardo is a guarantee of mankind's role as 'Safekeeper of the Human Genome'.

After elaborating on the issue of 'enframing', Heidegger goes on to question the notion of 'essence' as it is applied to modern technology. He makes it clear that the 'essence' of modern technology can never have the same connotations as the traditional notions of *genus* and *essentia* of the Platonic-Aristotelian school.[676] In fact, for Heidegger, it is precisely because these traditional notions only succeed in comprising 'all technological things' and nothing of the true essence of technology, that it became necessary to think of an alternative meaning of 'essence' as applied to modern technology that would go beyond the 'whatness' of a thing and give metaphysical significance to 'modern technology' that goes beyond the sense of *genus*.[677]

The first piece of the puzzle will lead him to the formulation of this new notion of 'essence' as applied to modern technology, Heidegger finds in the poem of Johann Peter Hebel, *Ghost on Kanderer Street*.[678] In the poem, the old German term *die Weserei* is used to signify 'city hall' with the connotations of 'community life' and 'village existence' that are constantly in play or 'essentially unfold'. *Die Weserei* is derived from the verb *wesen* that is typically translated as 'essence'. However, from *wesen*, Heidegger derives a nuanced meaning for the verb-form for which there is no counterpart in the English language and this is *wahren* that is normally translated as 'to endure'.[679] At this stage,

---

[676] Aristotle, *The Metaphysics,* trans. by Hugh Lawson-Tancred (London: Penguin Books, 2004), pp. 248–49.

[677] As the essence of a tree comprises those characteristics that are to be found in any tree, likewise the essence of technology employed in the same manner would have to be found in anything technological, be it a plough, kettle or any other technological device. For these reasons, Heidegger failed to comprehend how the traditional notion of essence could be applied to technology—hence his search for a new meaning of the term.

[678] Heidegger, 'The Question Concerning Technology', pp. 335–36.

[679] Ibid., p. 335.

Heidegger begins to use the terms 'essencing' and 'enduring' interchangeably. But he is not the first to use these two terms in this way because already Socrates and Plato had thought of 'essence' as 'something that unfolds essentially' in the sense of 'what endures or remains permanently' as, for example, the Platonic Idea of 'House'.[680] This notion of 'permanent enduring' leads Heidegger to his second piece of the puzzle to finding the true meaning of 'enframing'.

In the novel *Die Wunderlichen*, Johann Wolfgang von Goethe uses the word *fortgewahren* meaning 'to grant continuously' in place of the word *fortwahren* which means 'to endure continuously'.[681] Heidegger uses the different connotations of the two terms *fortgewahren* and *fortwahren* to establish a connection between the concept of 'enduring' as a quality of the 'wholeness' of a thing in the traditional sense that he derives from *fortwahren* and the concept of 'granting' that he derives from the term *forgewahren* which he then proposes as the basis of his novel interpretation of the 'essence/enframing' of modern technology:

> Only what is granted endures. What endures primally out of the earliest beginnings is what grants.[682]

But what is granted to humanity that endures? The answer is to be found in Holderlin's poem that speaks of the 'saving power' that grows 'where danger is'.[683] In other words, for Heidegger, modern technology's essential unfolding has within it and not outside of it, the saving power that humanity needs to build a free relationship with technology and so resist falling victim to it and become reduced to mere 'standing-reserve':

> The essential unfolding of technology threatens revealing, threatens it with the possibility that all revealing will be consumed in ordering and that everything will present itself only in the unconcealment of standing-reserve. Human activity can never directly counter this danger. Human achievement alone can never banish it. But human reflection can ponder the fact that all saving power must be of a higher 'essence than what is endangered, though at the same time kindred to it'.[684]

---

[680]   Ibid., pp. 335–36.

[681]   Ibid., p. 336.

[682]   *Die Wahlverwandtschaften*, quoted in Martin Heidegger, 'The Question Concerning Technology', in *Basic Writings* (London: Routledge, 2007), p. 336.

[683]   Heidegger, 'The Question Concerning Technology', p. 340.

[684]   Ibid., p. 339.

Thus 'enframing', for Heidegger, grants us the saving power to 'enter into a more original revealing and hence to experience the call of a more primal truth'.[685]

> For it is granting that first conveys to man that share in revealing which the coming-to-pass of revealing needs. As the one needed and used, man is given to belong to the coming-to-pass of truth. The granting that sends in one way or another into revealing is as such the saving power. For the saving power lets man see and enter into the highest dignity of his essence. This dignity lies in keeping watch over the unconcealment—and with it, from the first, the concealment—of all coming to presence on this earth.[686]

So against an orientation to the world that assumes that the world can and ought to be grasped and controlled through measurement and categorization, Heidegger offers mankind the possibility of tapping the redemptive quality of that which threatens us in the form of the saving power that can only have effect through human agency. This is the alternative mode of 'enframing' that Heidegger has been working towards and which, he believes, can save humanity from the dangers that are inherent in modern technology.

This is also the alternative mode of 'enframing' that can save the human genome from being reduced to its biological composition as a 'standing-reserve' or 'DNA repository' and from being seen primarily as an object of biotechnological manipulation. At this point in our study of Heidegger's thought it becomes clear that as 'Safekeepers of the Truth' we have the especial role of responsible stewardship of the human genome that is the embodiment of our self-identity as members of the human species. But we are also called upon to assume the responsible stewardship of biotechnology that will entail allowing the human genome to reveal itself on its own terms and not be 'challenged-forth' as a 'standing-reserve' waiting to be exploited. In other words, the human genome must not be seen as 'an object of technological manipulation' that exists only to satisfy our purposes but rather we should allow our purposes to be affected by and given creative expression by the qualities of the human genome itself. This is no easy task because, as Heidegger explains,

> The irresistibility of ordering and the restraint of the saving power draw past each other like the paths of two stars in the course of the heavens. But precisely this, their passing by, is the hidden side of nearness.

---

685 Ibid., p. 333.
686 Ibid., p. 337.

> When we look into the ambiguous essence of technology, we behold the constellation, the stellar course of the mystery.
>
> The question concerning technology is the question concerning the constellation in which revealing and concealing, in which the coming to presence of truth, comes to pass.[687]

'Looking into the constellation of truth' entails engaging in a constantly critical and questioning relationship with technology as it continually makes excursions into our daily life.[688] But primarily it must comprise a willingness to adopt a positive attitude of humility towards the physical world as it reveals itself on its own terms in the spirit of the classical concept of *techne* that was not used solely for technology but also for the fine arts that were characterized as a 'bringing-forth' of the true into the beautiful in the Aristotelian sense of *poiesis*. Naturally the same can be applied to the field of biotechnology and the human genome— we must engage into a constantly critical and questioning relationship with biotechnology that must be accompanied by a willingness to adopt a positive attitude towards the human genome. These goals can only ultimately be achieved by making the human genome the common heritage of mankind whence its exploitation will be guided by an international authority such as the International Human Genome Authority for and on behalf of all mankind. Allowing our purposes to be affected by and be given creative expression by the qualities of the human genome means that, as 'Safekeepers of the Human Genome', we must acknowledge the metaphysical reality of the genome as the embodiment of our humanness from which is derived our individual and species-identity.

Martin Heidegger pioneered a new way of thinking about technology that is not primarily concerned with the practical issues surrounding the use of particular technologies which form the basis of most contemporary debates on bioethics, both on a national and on an international level. These debates are normally between those who are in favour of using any new biotechnology as long as it is able to conquer disease and those who question certain biotechnologies such as cloning that are considered to be unethical for some reason or other. Instead, Heidegger's questioning is focussed on the ways of thinking that lie behind technology, including biotechnology. His concern lies with the essence of technology rather than with the function, utility and application of particular

---

[687]   Heidegger, 'The Question Concerning Technology', p. 338.
[688]   Ibid., p. 338.

technologies.[689] It follows that contemporary debates on bioethics should not be centred as they are on what biotechnologies should be allowed or not allowed but rather on the basic assumptions underlying the science that produces these biotechnologies![690] Peter Wilberg, the British philosopher and psychologist, argues that this science, which he refers to as Human Genomics, is purely reductionist in its approach to human beings because it reduces them to their biology and turns them into objects of biotechnology. This approach is solely concerned with scientific and instrumental conceptions of biotechnology and is totally blinded to the various effects and outcomes of biotechnologies on the fundamental issues of health and illness.[691] It is the result of the conditioning of man's orientation to the world by modern technology that hoodwinks him to all other modes of revealing outside of the technological disposition.[692]

The problem with Heidegger is that while he successfully revealed the essence of modern technology, he stopped at the point where he could have pursued his philosophical investigations into the nature of technology to argue in favour of a new ethics of responsibility which, as a matter of fact, was later brought into public discourse by Hans Jonas. Unlike Heidegger, when Arvid Pardo first proposed to make the deep seabed the common heritage of mankind, he did not stop at the proposal but went further and suggested to the international community the establishment of an international authority that would manage the deep seabed for and on behalf of all mankind, in the context of a New International Economic Order. In addressing the UN General Assembly, Pardo made it very clear that while, on the one hand, man's 'penetration of the deep could mark the beginning of the end for man, and indeed for life as we know it on this earth', at the same time, 'it could also be a unique opportunity to lay solid foundations for a peaceful and increasingly prosperous future for all peoples'.*[693]*

This is what makes Arvid Pardo a beacon of hope amidst the darkness and gloom that dominated international politics in the 1960s. This is what makes Arvid Pardo stand out from environmentalists, politicians and economists who

---

[689]   Zitzelsberger, 'Concerning Technology: Thinking with Heidegger', pp. 242–50.

[690]   Peter Wilberg, *Human Ontology or Human Genomics: Heidegger's Health Warning to Humanity*. <http://www.meaningofdepression.com/human%20Ontology.ppt> [accessed 20 January 2009]

[691]   Zitzelsberger, 'Concerning Technology: Thinking with Heidegger', pp. 242–50.

[692]   Craig A. Condella, *Overcoming the Destining of Technological Being*. Symposium: Humanity's Place in the Cosmos (6 November 2001). <http://www.fordham.edu/philosophy/fps/symposia/2001fall/condella.htm> [accessed 28 November 2008]

[693]   Pardo, *The Common Heritage of Mankind*, p. 2.

have spoken out against the squandering of Planet Earth, pointed fingers at others and stopped there! Arvid Pardo took the 'road less travelled' when he proposed the establishment of a new regime of international management for the resources of the deep seabed that would proscribe the unilateral exploitation of these resources by any nation or group.

In the 1960s, Pardo's concern was with the technological advances that made the exploitation of the deep seabed a tangible reality for those countries that chose to develop the necessary technology. These fears had not arisen before, even though the *Challenger* had found the cobalt and manganese nodules at the bottom of the deep seabed way back in 1873, because the technology to exploit these mineral resources did not exist at the time. In recent years, we have had a parallel situation when with the discovery of the molecular structure of DNA by Watson and Crick and the launching of the HGP, it became possible for some countries and groups such as pharmaceutical companies to exploit the human genome once they could develop the biotechnology to do so. The difference between the two situations is that while in the case of the deep seabed no serious attempt was ever made to develop the necessary technology to exploit these resources as it turned out that it was not cost-effective to do so, in the case of the human genome the biotechnology required to exploit it has been developed and continues to be developed at a very fast pace. This makes it all the more urgent to put an end to the commercialization of the human genome by re-routing the biotechnology train in such a manner that it better serves the interests of all mankind, considering that the human genome is, after all, our genome!

But as discussed earlier in our study, reaching through the genome with the HGP has had its share of problems ranging from squabbling over genetic patents, the issue of property rights in DNA, issues of privacy, the question of the anti-commons effect in biomedical research, and ultimately the uncertainty principle that is endemic to biotechnology. Most of these issues are related to the way the HGP has been conducted and it is our contention that most of the science behind the HGP is based on the wrong assumption that the human genome constitutes the Book of Life whose secret can be revealed by decoding its molecular constituents and structure. Peter Wilberg argues that this is equivalent to saying that a book, any book for that matter, can be understood by performing a number of tasks on the basic structure of the book itself such as scientifically analysing the ink marks on its paper, individuating a basic alphabet of these ink marks, cataloguing the different combinations and permutations and finally arriving at some form of explanation as to how these permutations produce sentences, paragraphs and chapters. What this approach to human genomics fails to acknowledge is that the ink marks on the book's pages are only the visible two-dimensional surface of an invisible multidimensional world of meaning! In other words, the text can only be understood because it is interpreted within the world of meaning it expresses. Applying the same to the human genome, it is an illusion to think for one moment that the meaning of human life or, metaphorically, the secret of the 'Holy Grail' can be known by deciphering the three-dimensional genetic structure of the Book of Life! Just as a chemical analysis of the ink marks on a page will not by itself reveal the meaning of the text, nor will the HGP by itself reveal the meaning of the human genome.[694]

This reflection will lead us to the next phase of our study where we will probe into the reasons behind the *enigma of health* that Hans-Georg Gadamer believes is made manifest when people prefer to ask someone 'Are you sick?' rather than 'Are you healthy?' and then proceed to demonstrate how the solution to this enigma can throw light on the role the human genome has in the field of human illness and health, that is, in the domain of medical treatment and its limits.

4.5   The Genome and the Enigma of Health

A student of Heidegger, Gadamer has focussed his attention on the way medical science is perceived by modern society which has itself been transformed by modern science. In his view, which he shares with Heidegger and Habermas among others, modern society's outlook on the phenomena of sickness and health has been greatly influenced by man's incessant drive to objectify the world with the ultimate aim of achieving complete technological mastery over nature.[695] During the past couple of decades, great advances have been made in the field of medical technology which unfortunately have tended to condition the thinking behind the way medical treatment is administered to patients. Just as Heidegger's River Rhine came to be viewed primarily as a hydroelectric plant as a result of the technological disposition, the human body came to be seen as 'little more than physicality that is calculable, predictable, and thus programmable to some extent'.[696] The same can be said about the human genome when it

---

694   Wilberg, *Human Ontology or Human Genomics*.
695   Fred Dallmayr, 'The Enigma of Health: Hans-Georg Gadamer at 100', *The Review of Politics*, 62 (2000) 327–50 (p. 327).
696   Zitzelsberger, 'Concerning Technology: Thinking with Heidegger', pp. 242–50.

is reduced to a 'DNA repository' of around 3 billion chemical base pairs whose identification is believed to be capable of revealing the secret of our humanness which will also become programmable in the future, through the marvels of biotechnological manipulation! This is a goal that, Gadamer remarks, contrasts sharply with the natural philosophy of antiquity that looked upon nature as a self-maintaining and self-restoring totality. Gadamer continually refers to Platos' *Phaedrus* with its holistic understanding of the human being as an essential part of the totality that is the world. In the dialogue, Socrates speaks of the need to 'know' the soul in order to 'heal' the body and the impossibility of healing the body and soul without knowing something about the 'unity of being itself' that can be interpreted as Heidegger's *Dasein*.[697] For Gadamer, as will be seen from our study, the practice of medical science is closely connected to a person's being and sense of life as it was with the Greeks with the focus of the art of healing on the restoration and maintenance of health. As modern medicine is primarily geared towards the understanding of disease and fighting illness, we tend to forget that our ultimate goal always remains the restoration of health:

> But the healing arts involve not only the successful struggle against illness but also the process of reconvalescence and, ultimately, care for health in the broadest sense.[698]

But it is within the perspective of modern science that Gadamer chooses to look upon the phenomena of sickness and health. In this context, he begins by distinguishing between the field of scientific medicine that is concerned with the knowledge of things in general and the art of healing that demands the concrete application of the knowledge of scientific medicine to particular cases. For Gadamer, it is only the first kind of knowledge that can be taught and learnt whereas the art of healing is something that no one learns from books but rather acquires through experience and the development of one's power of judgement.[699] The same can be said about human genomic knowledge and the biomedical application of this knowledge in the healthcare field. Knowing what kind of human genomic knowledge to pursue and discerning which of this knowledge should be applied in the biomedical fields are decisions that must be made in the best interests of all mankind. Again, it is our contention that by making the human

---

[697]   Dallmayr, 'The Enigma of Health', pp. 327–50.

[698]   Hans-Georg Gadamer, *The Enigma of Health: The Art of Healing in a Scientific Age* (California: Stanford University Press, 1996), p. 108.

[699]   Ibid., pp. 102–03.

genome the common heritage of mankind, we will be guaranteeing the total respect of these interests for and on behalf all mankind. More importantly, while
the common heritage of mankind will constitute the appropriate international
political model for human genome management, the choice of which human genomic knowledge is made applicable to the biomedical field must be based on
the model of the human person as proposed by Gadamer who, in his philosophical investigations on the art of healing, is able to re-discover the true significance of medical treatment by returning to the roots of this profession in the
annals of antiquity.

Similar views to those of Gadamer on this issue were expressed by Michael
Polanyi when he spoke about 'tacit knowledge' as the personal element involved
in a doctor's responsibility towards his patient. Whereas the rules of scientific
detachment require that we limit ourselves only to physical and chemical observations, such a stance does not allow us to get involved personally in the scientific endeavour.[700] Polanyi believes that any scientific research pursued in such
a detached and impersonal and materialistic way isolates itself from a human's
higher faculties and thereby restricts its power of discernment and understanding. On the other hand, a science which incorporates a personal component and
which is open to other branches of knowing allows us not only to understand the
true function of science but also our true function and purpose as persons.[701]
This is why it is so important to take into account metaphysical considerations
of the human genome. Like Philippa Foot[702] and Iris Murdoch[703], we believe
that a metaphysical account of human nature, including the human genome, is
necessary if we are to apply human genomic knowledge to biomedical science.
Only a human genomic metaphysics will ensure that our ethical thinking on biomedical issues will not slide to a reductionist subjectivism that will deny the
human genome its true essential nature. Considering that as of January 2009,
over 3 million genome-related patent applications have been filed on genes, gene
fragments, SNPs,[704] gene tests, proteins and stem cells, the need to fight against

---

[700] Michael Polanyi, *Knowing and Being* (London: Routledge & Kegan, 1969), p. 123.

[701] Polanyi, *The Tacit Dimension*, pp. 24–25.

[702] Philippa Foot, *Natural Goodness* (Oxford: Oxford University Press, 2001).

[703] Iris Murdoch, *Sovereignty of Good* (London: Routledge, 2001).

[704] Single Nucleotide Polymorphisms are DNA sequence variations that occur when a single nucleotide in the genome sequence is altered. Many SNPs have no effect on cell function but
scientists believe that others could predispose people to disease or influence their response to

this fragmentation of the human genome becomes more urgent than ever. Already there are several gatekeeper-patents that are exercising excessive control over the biomedical benefits of human genome research—making the human genome the common heritage of mankind is the most effective way of fighting against the fragmentation of the human genome in the interests of all mankind.

Going back to the example of a doctor about to perform a patient's diagnosis, 'tacit knowledge' is that unaccountable and inarticulate component of knowledge that makes us seem to know more than we actually know![705] Like the child of ten who is able to ride a bicycle without being able to state the rules governing turning, balance, speed and the angle of disequilibrium, tacit knowing is the fundamental power of the mind that not only creates and lends meaning to explicit knowing but also controls it. Gestalt psychology explains this phenomenon by demonstrating how we recognize a face by integrating its particulars impressed in our brain into a comprehensive entity.[706] Integration occurs as we shift our attention from the parts to the whole. And the whole is not simply a sum of parts because the parts take on a different meaning in the whole. When we see a whole, we see the individual parts differently from the way we see them in isolation. There is an active shaping of experience that happens within us, that transforms the parts themselves even as it transforms the parts into a comprehensive entity. The same happens when we attend only subsidiarily to the two-dimensional words in a text in order to permit tacit integration and understand the multidimensional meanings that are conveyed through the text.[707] So tacit knowing is a dynamic process that grows increasingly meaningful with time and experience.

It is maybe for this reason, because a purely objective position does not allow a doctor to participate personally in his rapport with a patient, that it has proved necessary to coin the phrase 'quality of life' in the field of medical care.[708] This was done, Gadamer believes, with the purpose of ensuring that the patient's needs and desires remain at the heart of professional medical care and that he or she is not reduced to a [human] machine requiring only technical assistance in order to resume its proper functions. And one of the skills acquired

---

a drug. This makes SNPs of great value for biomedical research and for developing pharmaceutical products or medical diagnostics.

[705]   Polanyi, *The Tacit Dimension*, p. 4.
[706]   Ibid., p. 6.
[707]   Mark T. Mitchell, *Michael Polanyi* (Delaware: ISI Books, 2006), pp. 73–74.
[708]   Gadamer, *Enigma of Health*, p. 104.

in the art of healing, through lived human experience, is the ability to judge the ways and means how medical science can be made to contribute to a patient's 'quality of life'. This expression, for Gadamer, reveals,

> ...a fundamental and immemorial human recognition that each of us has to 'lead' our own lives and that we must decide for ourselves how we are going to live.[709]

But the problem that Gadamer raises is whether medical science can be more appropriately defined as the 'science of illness' or the 'science of health'. On the one hand, it is illness that 'objectifies' itself, confronting us as something opposed to us and forcing itself upon us. So when we are sick we talk of our illness as a 'case of illness'. Gadamer refers to the German word for 'case' that is '*fall*' which is a word that originates from the game of dice and refers to the role which 'falls' to a noun within a sentence. Likewise, an illness is something that 'befalls' or 'falls' to us. The Greek word for 'symptom' has a very close meaning to the German word for 'fall' as it is used to refer to the conspicuous features that become manifest when an illness 'befalls' us.[710] On the other hand, health, unlike illness, escapes objectification because it does not really actually present itself to us, argues Gadamer.[711] There is a real mystery in the hidden character of health that makes it absurd to ask someone, 'Are you healthy?'. According to Gadamer, it is because health is a condition of inner accord and of harmony with oneself that it defies measurement and standardization.[712] He challenges the notion that health can be technically engineered or made because it defies the project of mastery over nature that is the goal of modern medical science.[713] And it is precisely for this reason that the human genome could never be the Holy Grail of biology with the answers to all problems of ill health that many imagine it to be. Many were the people who were misguided in their projections for the future of medical health when they thought that once the identification of the thousands of human genes that made up the human genome was complete then we would be able to take a proactive stand in the face of medical illness and through genetic intervention be able to eradicate a disease before it begins to manifest its symptoms.

---

[709] Ibid.
[710] Gadamer, *Enigma of Health*, p. 107.
[711] Ibid.
[712] Ibid., pp. 107–8.
[713] Ibid.

For Gadamer, contrary to what medical science may aspire to achieve, health will never be the product of manipulation or forceful intervention as epitomized in Aldous Huxley's *Brave New World*[714] that depicts human life seven centuries from now when with genetic manipulation, psychoactive drugs, hypnopaedia and high-tech amusements, disease is totally eliminated together with aggression, war, anxiety, suffering, guilt and grief.[715] *Brave New World* anticipates the biomedical project of medical science to preserve and prolong bodily life at the expense of stripping human life of much of its dignity. Aldous Huxley managed to portray in a brilliant way how progress can become tragedy when one individual, the 'Savage', who is a human being bred by natural means, dares confront the 'Controller', Mustapha Mond:

> 'But I don't want comfort. I want God, I want poetry, I want real danger, I want freedom, I want goodness, I want sin'.
> 'In fact', said the Savage defiantly, 'I'm claiming the right to be unhappy'.
> 'Not to mention the right to grow old and ugly, and impotent; the right to have syphilis and cancer; the right to have too little to eat; the right to be lousy; the right to live in constant apprehension of what may happen tomorrow; the right to catch typhoid; the right to be tortured by unspeakable pains of every kind'.[716]

This is a confrontation between, on the one hand, the drug 'soma'[717] that is a single-chemical combination of many of today's drugs' effects and a symbol for the powerful influence of science and technology on society and, on the other hand, the humanness of the Savage that symbolizes Gadamer's understanding of health as something that each and every one of us must take care of through the way we choose to lead our lives:

> What is important is to recognize the other in their otherness, as opposed, for example, to the tendency towards standardization promoted by modern technology, the autocratic control of education by school authorities or the blind insistence on authority by a teacher or a father. Only by means of such recognition can we hope to provide genuine guidance which helps the other to find their own independent way. Treatment always involves also a certain granting of freedom.[718]

---

714   Aldous Huxley, *Brave New World* (London: Flamingo, 1994).
715   Kass, *Life, Liberty and the Defence of Dignity*, p. 5.
716   Huxley, *Brave New World*, p. 219.
717   In Aldous Huxley's Brave New World, soma is a drug that provides an easy escape from the hassles of daily life and is used by the government as a method of control through pleasure.
718   Gadamer, *Enigma of Health*, p. 109.

The confrontation is also between those who believe that biology alone can explain illness and health and those who believe that biology cannot ignore metaphysical considerations about life and reality. In a sense it is a confrontation between biotechnological humanism that rejects any form of human genomic metaphysics and transcendental humanism that looks upon the human genome as being the true essence of human nature with external influences considered to be mere accidental occasions. *Brave New World* is obviously a work of science fiction but the likeness between Huxley's fictional world and our own world are frankly disquieting when we consider the great advances that have been made in the past years in the area of biotechnology[719] and its application to many of the external influences of human nature rather than its true essential nature.

4.6 The Art of Healing as an Epiphany for Biotechnology

Biotechnological humanism is a product of modern technology and it will lead to human debasement rather than fulfilment. By reflecting on the especial role that the doctor has with his patient, Gadamer paves the way for a road that will put biotechnology at the service of compassionate humaneness that will not allow the achievement of perfected bodies at the price of flattened souls![720] He proceeds on this path by reflecting on that 'inner proportion or inner correspondence that cannot be measured and yet must always be taken into account'.[721]

First he explains the role of the doctor that must be one of caring for the patient in such a manner that he can verify the patient's own subjective localization or experience of pain. He refers to the German word, *behandeln,* which is equivalent to the Latin word *palpare,* meaning 'with the hand' or *palpus.*[722] He then proceeds to explain that the living use of the term *behandeln* goes beyond the specific domain of medicine because everyone, irrespective of his profession in life, is called to treat others correctly by not forcing ourselves on them or compelling them to accept things or do things against their own will. According to Gadamer, this will only not happen when we choose to recognize 'the other in their otherness'.[723] In the doctor-patient relationship, the doctor will choose not to impose himself on his patient when he responsibly undertakes to

---

[719] Kass, *Life, Liberty and the Defence of Dignity*, p. 6.
[720] Ibid., p. 134.
[721] Gadamer, *Enigma of Health*, p. 108.
[722] Ibid.
[723] Ibid., p. 109.

use his medical expertise to help the patient recover from his illness but at the same time recognizing in the patient, the freedom to find his own, independent way. This requires that the doctor's skill to cure illness must not only prove effective in relieving the patient of the symptoms of his illness but, more importantly, must be accepted by the patient who is ill. So it is not a question of simply filling out a prescription and handing it to the patient, nor is it a question of 'getting rid of it' as, comments Gadamer, surgeons are wont to say to a patient who is about to undergo surgery.[724] This way of talking tends to look upon the illness of a patient as having a separate existence from him and which the doctor must destroy. But this is not the real task of the doctor, according to Gadamer. To him, doctors should not really be expected to 'make' or 'do' anything—rather they should humbly contribute towards guiding health in a certain manner so as to help the patient get better![725] Health, to Gadamer is a general feeling of well-being and,

> …it shows itself above all where such a feeling of well-being means we are open to new things, ready to embark on new enterprises and, forgetful of ourselves, scarcely notice the demands and strains which are put on us.[726]

Given that the disruption of health that normally necessitates treatment of a patient by a doctor puts the patient in an unequal relationship with the doctor, it is vital that the patient is free to discuss his or her illness with the doctor because dialogue and discussion serve to humanize the inequality of the doctor-patient relationship which, according to Gadamer, remains one of the most difficult challenges that confront human beings. The disruption of health brings with it a disturbance in one's equilibrium that must perforce be redressed by applying a counterforce which can easily cause a new loss of equilibrium! Medical treatment will act as this counterforce in the disruption of health but care must be taken so as not to induce a new imbalance through, for example, unnecessary prescriptions. Gadamer explains the delicate balance that must be maintained by the medical practitioner in dialogue with his patient by referring to the words of Rilke who in the *Duino Elegies* speaks of how, 'The permanently too little springs over into the empty too much'.[727] So every effort must be made for the

---

[724]   Ibid., p. 110.
[725]   Gadamer, *Enigma of Health*, p. 109.
[726]   Ibid., p. 112.
[727]   Ibid., p. 114.

doctor to discern exactly the right moment and the right dosage when treating a patient.[728] The same concerns have been expressed by Daniel Callahan, one of the founders of bioethics who has argued in favour of a healthcare system that helps the patient cope with the failings of the body rather than one that is unilaterally focussed on the conquering of disease and the extension of life at all costs.[729]

And, according to Gadamer, here lies the enigmatic character of health for it is none other than 'the rhythm of life, a permanent process in which equilibrium re-establishes itself'. He speaks of the three processes of breathing, digesting and sleeping which are three rhythmic phenomena that help to produce vitality, refreshment and the restoration of energy.[730] Although these rhythmic functions are not under our control, they constitute an integral part of ourselves and in fact, sustain us. But these phenomena have little to do with the consumption of medicines or the conscious effort to control them.[731]

Quoting a famous saying of Heraclitus, 'the harmony which is hidden is always stronger than that which is revealed', which is taken by Gadamer to refer to the harmonious balance of the 'humours' in ancient medicine, Gadamer explains that,

> The harmony of health only displays its real strength where it does not leave us numbed and deadened, that disturbing effect revealed or produced by persisting pain or the debilitating rush of intoxication.[732]

To Gadamer, therefore, medical treatment must be related to the 'totality' of the human person and its methods and goals should be concerned with the hidden harmony that must be constantly recovered and in which is discovered both the miracle of reconvalescence and the mystery of health. Gadamer reminds us that we are part of nature and it is in fact this nature within us that, together with the self-sustaining organic defence mechanism of our bodies, is able to sustain our 'inner' equilibrium which is what constitutes life. It follows that we should constantly remind ourselves that we can only oppose nature through being part of nature ourselves and through being sustained by nature lest we forget that both

---

[728]   Ibid.
[729]   Daniel Callahan, as quoted by Green in *Babies by Design*, pp. 3–4.
[730]   Gadamer, *Enigma of Health*, p. 114.
[731]   Ibid., p. 115.
[732]   Ibid., pp. 115–16.

the doctor and patient must together acknowledge the role of nature if successful recovery is to be accomplished.[733]

Before proceeding further, it must be said that stem cell therapies may, in the future, appear to provide a partial solution to Gadamer's *enigma of health* when, in virtue of their ability to differentiate into healthy mature cells, they can be used to replace damaged or diseased cells without necessitating the removal of these diseased cells through surgery or radiation. In other words, stem cell therapy can use the natural powers of the body to regenerate itself without the need of using external force on the body to excise the diseased cells.[734] This kind of medical science remains a possibility in the future because even though researchers have developed the science to regenerate the blood cells necessary to treat a leukaemia patient, for example, chemotherapy or radiation must be used first to destroy the cancerous cells in the blood. The problem is that since chemotherapy and radiation do not discriminate between healthy and diseased cells, they also destroy healthy blood cells and the stem cells that produce them. It is the bone marrow that is transfused into the patient that subsequently regenerates the required cells.[735] The fact that scientists have still not found a way around the use of chemotherapy or radiation that kill both healthy and cancerous cells means that research in this field is still in its infancy. This makes it even more important that the patent system is not allowed to create obstacles in the path of those researchers who are working towards trying to overcome these problems. This can only be avoided by (i) making the human genome the common heritage of mankind, (ii) overhauling the patent system by putting community rights before individual rights and (iii) by retrieving a science of the human genome that leaves no space for reductively biological considerations.

4.7   The Permanent Limitations of Biology

Medical practice must make definitive decisions about life and death based on current scientific knowledge that, by its very nature, remains incomplete and temporary. And modernity has systematically tended to restrict what counts as real knowledge to only that which can be known by scientific experiment. As a direct result of this reductive approach to knowledge, medical practice is forced to treat current scientific knowledge as if it had the final word on everything.

---

[733]   Ibid., p. 116.
[734]   Russell Kkorobkin, *Stem Cell Century: Law and Policy for a Breakthrough Technology* (New Haven: Yale University Press, 2007), p. 20.
[735]   Ibid., p. 22.

Gadamer blames the metaphysical agnosticism of modernity for the current situation that insists on explaining illness and health in purely physiological or neurophysiologic terms. But according to Gadamer, metaphysics is essential for reflecting on the meaning of health and such a need is made manifest when doctors refuse to subsume their patients under general scientific schemata and persist in maintaining a 'special relationship' with their patients, believing, as the Greek physicians of antiquity did, that one cannot treat the body without concomitantly treating the soul. The *manner* in which doctors practice the art of healing today has changed significantly from the way it was practised in classical times but the *matter* that concerns medical practice, namely the patient's whole being has not changed and medical science on its own is simply inadequate to deal with questions of life and reality that pertain more to metaphysics. Gadamer's conclusion is that in order to understand the question of health, what is needed is metaphysics rather than biology. And as the human genome has acquired such a pivotal role in current debates about healthcare issues, it is imperative that metaphysical considerations about life and reality are not ignored because they do not fit into the general schemata of medical science. Progress must not be achieved at the expense of flattened and soulless human genomes that will result in human debasement rather than fulfilment. This is the challenge of modern bioethical thinking, that it brings back into the field of biotechnology metaphysical considerations that are at the heart of our self-understanding as a species with the special responsibility of stewardship for and on behalf of all life on earth. For Gadamer, the health of society is a reflection of the health of the individual! It follows that in discussing issues of health and illness the philosopher must insist on the urgent need to make the human genome the centre of all bioethical thinking by preserving its identity as the soul of humankind. Making the human genome the common heritage of mankind in the Pardosian understanding of the term will ensure that it will never become the object of complete mastery by biotechnology. In the spirit of Arvid Pardo's original intentions in proposing to make the deep seabed the common heritage of mankind, the human genome should also not be made subject to exploitation or use if such activity may lead to flattened modes of existence for mankind.

4.8 Ethics for Biotechnology

A theory of ethics for the technological age was first proposed by Hans Jonas when he became acutely aware of how modern technology had disturbed the balance between humanity and nature in ways that were 'long-range, cumulative, irreversible and planetary in scale'.[736] His position rejected the nihilism of his teacher Heidegger and before him Nietzsche. Jonas argued in favour of universal human values and responsibilities that were binding on every human being irrespective of race, culture or religion. Like Gadamer and Habermas, Jonas was trained in the philosophical school of Heidegger and like them, he continued to be influenced by the master's mode of inquiry while at the same time abandoning many of his values.

The driving force behind Jonas' philosophy is the selfish and dangerous misuse of technology that is a threat to the conditions of human life for future generations and also undermines humanity's foundations within the natural world and the globe. Technology, together with the science that makes it possible, gives mankind a new kind of power that can have consequences that reach far into the future. This means that the actions that we take today can affect the lives of millions of people in the future notwithstanding the fact that these same people have no say in the decisions we make for them. It is precisely for these reasons that Jonas argues in favour of a new dimension of ethical responsibility, never dreamt of before, that must comprise concern for the global condition of human life together with the future existence of the human species.[737] Traditional ethics presumed that the effects of our actions were limited to the here and now and so the focus was prevalently on 'neighbourhood ethics'.[738] It is precisely for the 'time dimension' that Jonas includes in his ethical thinking that his philosophical investigations into the nature of modern technology which have also included biotechnology are so relevant to our discourse on making the human genome the common heritage of mankind. The political and ethical implications of the concept of common heritage of mankind are not time barred but on the contrary they must have, as their main object of concern, the well-being of future generations whose lives can be adversely affected by policy decisions taken by preceding generations. The philosophical concerns of Hans Jonas can be undoubtedly met by making the human genome the common heritage of mankind when the exploitation of the human genome will be carried out for and on behalf of all mankind for exclusively peaceful purposes. More importantly, the concept also contemplates the non-exploitation of the human genome if it is deemed to be in the best interests of all mankind.

---

[736]   Jonas, *Imperative of Responsibility*, p. 168.
[737]   Ibid., pp. 1–24.
[738]   Jonas, *Philosophical Essays*, p. 7.

Without doubt, modern technology has been accompanied with the development of new branches of ethics in various new academic fields such as biomedical ethics, computer ethics and environmental ethics. In these new disciplines, the ethical issues that are being pursued differ depending on the specific interests of each particular field. Still, there are two main concerns that are common to all these new applications of ethics and these are (i) the question of social justice in relation to the fair distribution of the benefits derived from these new technological applications and (ii) the question of risks and uncertainties that often accompany modern technology and biotechnology in particular. There are potential risks, for example, in Intracytoplasmic Sperm Injection (ICSI) that is believed to cause sterility in children conceived by this method of artificial reproduction, and in Xenotransplantation that is known to result in a number of new and uncontrollable diseases. There are also problems with human cloning by nuclear transfer as data obtained from the same procedure applied on animals has shown us. But the *hell scenario* remains associated with germline interventions intended to modify the human genome that can cause irreversible and catastrophic harm to future generations.

4.9 The Tragedy of Biotechnology

The tragedy that followed the genetic intervention on children carrying the X-SCID genetic disorder is a constant reminder of the serious risks involved in these new biotechnologies. In 2000, researchers from the Necker Hospital for Sick Children in Paris attempted a new form of genetic intervention with X-SCID children who had not responded to bone marrow therapy. The researchers removed a sample of blood from each child and after exposing the cells to a retrovirous that was genetically altered to carry a corrected DNA sequence for the IL 2R9 gene, the genetically modified blood cells were transfused back into each child and allowed to multiply. In a short time, nine out of the twelve children treated were producing healthy immune cells that could fight off infections. The researchers had successfully replaced the defective IL 2R9 gene that was not coding for the necessary proteins to make the interleukin-2 receptor that is needed for a proper functioning of the immune system. But things were not as they seemed because within one year of the genetic intervention, two of the ten children developed leukaemia with another child contracting the condition a year later. Tests showed that the corrected DNA sequence for the required IL 2R9 gene had inadvertently coded for leukaemia as when it was inserted in the genome, it 'placed' itself in an area that normally activated a leukaemia-connected gene. The possibility of this actually happening was there from the beginning but researchers considered it a very small risk and so they took a chance. From the very beginning researchers knew that there was a problem with the way corrected gene sequences integrated with the DNA sequences of the human genome into which they are introduced. The reason is that the corrected gene simply lodges itself anywhere among the 3 billion chemical nucleotides of the genome and, normally, is able to correct the defective gene it was introduced to remedy, without difficulty, irrespective of its location in the genome. But, and there is often a *but* in biotechnology, 'insertional mutagenesis' occurs which results in the corrector gene disrupting the normal functioning of some genes that were not meant to be targeted by it. The result is an artificially induced coding of otherwise normal genes as happened in the case of the X-SCID kids when the corrector gene for the IL 2R9 receptor mistakenly activated a leukaemia-connected gene! The result has become a well-known fact which must not be passed over as an unfortunate incident, even though it must be said that the children affected were eventually successfully treated for leukaemia with only one fatality among the ten children who probably would have succumbed to X-SCID if the child did not undergo genetic therapy.[739]

Hans Jonas established himself as a powerful intellectual figure when as a path breaker he brought into public discourse new concerns about the ethics of responsibility in relation to modern technology that have served as beacons in the complex and multifaceted public debate that has ensued after Martin Heidegger first subjected technology to philosophical scrutiny. Concerned about the catastrophic results that can ensue from biotechnological interventions of the kind discussed above, Jonas argued in favour of giving precedence to 'bad prognosis' over 'good prognosis'.[740] To him there is only one possible way open to us as a solution to the uncertainty that is inherent in the biotechnological mode of doing and this is to exercise *caution* in the face of the possible harmful effects that can be produced by biotechnology:

---

[739]   Green, *Babies by Design*, pp. 34–35.
[740]   Jonas, *The Imperative of Responsibility*, p. 31.

The principle for the treatment of uncertainty is itself not uncertain at all, and it binds us unconditionally—that is, not just as an advice of moral prudence but as an unqualified command—provided we accept the responsibility for what will be. Under such responsibility, caution, otherwise a peripheral matter of our discretion becomes the core of moral action.[741]

Jonas' interpretation of responsibility takes the form of a number of ethical principles that are at the basis of his cautionary approach to biotechnology. The first of these principles is the notion of the *heuristics of fear* by which Jonas intends that when there is doubt as to the possible outcome of a decision, one should always opt for the safer option.[742] The second is an admonition to always avoid any sort of action that might destroy the basis for future possibilities of human life. The third is an injunction to always include, in our present choices, the future integrity of human beings as an object of our concern.[743]

Already Jonas had realized that biotechnology was different from all other forms of technology because in biotechnological engineering, man is both the subject and the object of the technology. This was one of the main features of modern technology to which Martin Heidegger alerted the philosophical community in his *The Questioning Concerning Technology*. The metaphysical implications of this unique characteristic of biotechnology cannot be overestimated. It must be borne in mind when considering the human genome as the common heritage of mankind because great caution must be employed so as not to underestimate the extent to which humankind can become itself the direct object of technological mastery.

Another feature that distinguishes biotechnology from other forms of modern technology is the fact that the object of biological enquiry is living material and/or life forms that are either discovered in nature or invented after being made subject to modification by biological engineering. With biotechnology, therefore, the object of technological control is not an artefact that is made from non-living material but actual 'living entities' and for this reason, the products of biotechnological engineering are very difficult to predict.[744] When speaking about cloning, Professor Stuart Newman, from the New York Medical College, warned of the dangers that accompany biological interventions:

---

[741]   Ibid., p. 38.
[742]   Ibid., pp. 26–27.
[743]   Jonas, *Philosophical Essays*, pp. 13–14.
[744]   Ibid., p. 143.

All scientists know that when you do a biological experiment it sometimes works and sometimes doesn't. If it works 70–80% of the time you are really lucky.[745]

But again, even though the experiment may appear to be successful, it will take a couple of generations before you can ascertain the fact. Newman takes as an example the germline modification of an animal that despite the animal appearing to be normal in all respects, its offspring may develop cancer at forty times the normal rate![746]

As a result, a number of problems endemic to biotechnology cannot be ignored as has been wisely advised by Paul Ramsey:

> For the biological engineer, who has to take over, 'sight-unseen', the untold complexity of the given determinants with their self-functioning dynamics, the number of unknowns in the design is immense. To them he must commit his contributory share in the totality of causes. Prediction of its fate is thus reduced to guessing, planning—to gambling. The intended redesigning or modification or improvement is in fact an 'experiment' and one with so long a run—at least in the genetic field—that its outcome (if identifiable at all) lies normally beyond the purview of the experimenter himself.[747]

With other forms of technological engineering, the properties of the engineered product can normally be predicted with accuracy. The computer engineer, to take an example, builds his product starting from separate components that he puts together according to a specific programme or blueprint that he designs himself. But with biotechnology the bio-engineer does not work with a blueprint because the blueprint is the biological system itself that develops and functions within a set of boundary conditions that are determined by a controlling-principle that is not reducible to physical-chemical mechanisms.[748]

It is precisely because human engineering operates on the 'original' itself rather than 'construct' that Jonas cautions us to consider well the consequences of human engineering before using it. According to Jonas, when the predictability of a certain application of biotechnological engineering is in question because of the number of unknowns involved, wisdom may dictate that the best course of action would be to refrain from pursuing such a line of investigation that is fraught with uncertainty. Referring to Pascal's famous wager that it is

---

[745]   Stuart Newman, *The Role of Genetic Reductionism in Biocolonialism*, quoted in Mckibben, *Enough: Staying Human in an Engineered Age*, p. 41.

[746]   Ibid.

[747]   Jonas, *Philosophical Essays*, p. 143.

[748]   Ibid., p. 144.

better to 'bet' in favour of the existence of God as the odds in favour of believing are far superior to those in favour of not-believing since eternal happiness is always preferable to eternal damnation, Jonas prefers to err on the side of caution rather than on the side of negligence.[749]

The *Washington Post* reporter, Joel Garreau has made two interesting remarks in his book, *Radical Evolution,* on the question of biotechnology, that do not originate from the biotechnical or bioethical camp. The first remark concerns an article published in *Wired Magazine* by Bill Joy, one of the founders of the Information Age, who has warned his readers about the catastrophic consequences that biological engineering can have on the human species if the biotechnological revolution is allowed to develop and progress without any form of control or regulation. Particularly, Joy has expressed concern about the possibility of bio-engineers taking natural evolution into their own hands and creating, in the laboratory, a number of subhuman species that would not possess the same human capabilities with which natural evolution has endowed natural mankind. Although many would find such a suggestion as being 'offensive, grotesque, revolting, repugnant and repulsive', to quote the words of Leon Kass,[750] there are other intellectuals such as Michael Tooley who have pronounced that they find no moral objection to the use of cloning to produce mindless organ banks so that if an individual needs a heart transplant, the clone's heart can be used without any fear of organ rejection! Tooley considers this use of human cloning as beneficial to society as long as the clones are not persons, hence the requirement that they be 'mindless'![751] But, as Garreau notes, this takes us back to the point raised by Bill Joy that maybe, we should not even consider creating the clones in the first place.[752]

The second remark concerns the science fiction series *Star Trek* that was the creation of Gene Roddenberry and that has captured the imagination of millions of spectators all over the world, including Bill Joy. Many books have been written on *Star Trek* ranging from the *Physics of Star Trek*[753] of Lawrence

---

[749]   Jonas, *Imperative of Responsibility*, p. 37.

[750]   Leon R. Kass and James Q. Wilson, *The Ethics of Human Cloning* (Washington D.C.: AEI Press, 1998), p. 17.

[751]   James M. Humber and Robert F. Almeder (eds.), *Human Cloning* (Totwa: Humania Press, 1998).

[752]   Joel Garreau, *Radical Evolution: The Promise and Peril of Enhancing our Minds, our Bodies— and What it Means to Be Human* (New York: Doubleday, 2004), pp. 135–48.

[753]   Lawrence Krauss, *The Physics of Star Trek* (London: Flamingo, 1997).

Krauss with a foreword by Stephen Hawking to the *Ethics of Star Trek*[754] by Judith Barard. Basically *Star Trek* is about humans exploring the cosmos and making first contact with people from different planets. In meeting with these peoples, some more intelligent and others less intelligent than us, the people of Earth were to follow a strict moral code that was referred to by all as the Prime Directive:

> As the right of each sentient species to live in accordance with its normal cultural evolution is considered sacred, no Star fleet personnel may interfere with the healthy development of alien life and culture. Such interference includes the introduction of superior knowledge, strength, or technology to a world whose society is incapable of handling such advantages wisely. Star Fleet personnel may not violate this Prime Directive, even to save their lives and/or their ship unless they are acting to right an earlier violation or an accidental contamination of said culture. This directive takes precedence over any and all other considerations, and carries with it the highest moral obligation.[755]

This Directive is envisaging a future where ethical human beings will be respectful of the particular stage of natural evolution that the peoples of the different planet would have reached. On this Garreau makes two comments, one on the incredible appeal that the ethical implications of the Directive had on Bill Joy and two on the possibility that humans may already be violating the Prime Directive on their home planet.[756]

Bill Joy called for the relinquishment of those technologies that posed a serious threat to mankind. The Prime Directive forbade the introduction of any technology to a society that was incapable of handling the advantages it offered. Hans Jonas and Arvid Pardo advocated the relinquishment of technology if this technology was bound to result in catastrophic consequences for mankind. On the one hand, Hans Jonas admonished us to refrain from pursuing biotechnological engineering if it was deemed wise not to do so. On the other hand, Arvid Pardo admonished the UN General Assembly to claim the deep seabed as the common heritage of mankind and challenged the international community to reinvent the *res communis* regime of public property by suggesting that the responsible stewardship of these resources may require that we refrain from exploiting them if it is deemed wise not to do so, in the interests of all mankind, especially future generations.

---

[754]   Judith Barard, *The Ethics of Star Trek* (New York: Perennial, 2000).
[755]   Garreau, *Radical Evolution*, p. 141.
[756]   Ibid.

Bill McKibben has proposed two challenges for the world of today that we can make our own, namely (i) that we have the courage to regulate technological innovation in order that we remain 'more or less human'[757] and (ii) that we allow the rush of technological innovation that has marked the past 500 years to slow down![758] Making the human genome the common heritage of mankind is one way of regulating biotechnological innovation and imposing a moratorium on genetic patents could be the first step towards building the necessary framework to have the exploitation of the human genome managed by an international authority for and on behalf of all mankind.

4.10 Re-Thinking Biotechnology with the Human Genome as Common Heritage of Mankind

More recently, Jurgen Habermas has echoed the words of Hans Jonas when he predicted catastrophic consequences on the human species, as a result of biological engineering, if the biotechnological revolution is allowed to develop and progress without any regulation as is the case at the moment. Jurgen Habermas argues for an unmanipulated genetic heritage because any such genetic manipulation will touch the core of our identity as human beings. According to Habermas, human beings have come to understand themselves in certain determined ways that cannot be simply brushed away by modern science that sees biotechnology as the ultimate achievement of man. Fundamental to Habermas' thought is the belief that human beings have traditionally understood themselves as ethically free individuals who are authors of their own lives and who approach other human beings with the expectation that they too are authors of their own lives![759] On the basis of this fundamental precept, societal integration has been accompanied with the establishment of norms that are meant to respect an individual's autonomy and put a limit on an individual's imposition on others.

The problem for Habermas is that any form of genetic manipulation of the human genome such as, for example, the genetic programming of human beings will create a divide within the human species that puts on one side the genetic programmers, and on the other side, the genetically programmed:

---

[757]   McKibben, *Enough: Staying Human in an Engineered Age*, p. 197.
[758]   Ibid., p. 198.
[759]   Ibid., p. 33.

> The program designer carries out a one-sided act for which there can be no well-founded assumption of consent, disposing over the genetic factors of another in the paternalistic intention of setting the course, in relevant respects, of the life history of the dependent person. The latter may interpret, but not revise or undo this intention. The consequences are irreversible because the paternalistic intention is laid down in a disarming genetic program instead of being communicatively mediated by a socializing practice which can be subjected to reappraisal by the person 'raised'.[760]

If we take Michael Tooley's proposal for cloning human beings as an example, we will have the cloners or bio-engineers on one side and the clones or mindless organ banks on the other side. C.S. Lewis managed to capture Habermas' thought in his essay of 1944, *The Abolition of Man*:

> Man's conquest of Nature, if the dreams of some scientific planners are realized, means the rule of a few hundreds of men over billions upon billions of men.[761]

In order to avoid the emergence of this divide, Habermas believes that the 'inalienable normative conceptions of societal integration' must be safeguarded because they are at the basis of the 'species-ethic' that has its roots in our anthropological self-understanding as a species. And it is in fact this 'species-ethic' that underpins Habermas' preoccupation with biotechnological applications that threaten to undermine our self-referentiality as a human species.

There are many applications of biotechnology that, according to Habermas, are violating our dignity as human persons. For one, he is totally against the use of biotechnology to selectively modify and/or engineer specific genetic traits for purely enhancement purposes. Even the genetic research that goes into applying biotechnology to the bio-engineering of desired characteristics is problematic to Habermas because, he believes, this pioneering 'concept biotechnology' can overshadow ordinary genetic research for medical use that is primarily focussed on therapeutic intervention rather than on biotechnical enhancements of the human body.[762] It seems to Habermas that through the use of biotechnology, man is losing respect for the 'given' or what comes by nature, because he has become fascinated with what he can 'make' or what is manufactured. At the same time man is not giving due consideration to the possibility that individuals that are genetically enhanced may no longer see themselves as 'undivided authors' of their own lives because of the biotechnical interventions to which they were

---

[760] Habermas, *The Future of Human Nature*, 2005, p. 64.
[761] Lewis, *Abolition of Man*, p. 58.
[762] Habermas, *The Future of Human Nature*, 2005, p. 28.

made subject. This could also lead to a situation where these individuals may be perceived as bioengineered 'augments' with the result that they may experience interpersonal relationships that are no longer characterized by the 'egalitarian premises of morality and law'. At this point, argues Habermas, the biotechnology developed by individuals who are 'authors of their own life history' begins to undermine this very feature of our humanity![763]

When Hans Jonas wrote *The Imperative of Responsibility* in 1979, the first positive reactions to the book came from the political camp with Helmut Schmidt and Hans-Dietrich Genscher losing no time in making their views publicly known. The political interest in his philosophical work put Jonas in the unique position of being able to exert political influence because of his philosophical insights![764] Jurgen Habermas was able to attain a similar political influence on issues of bioethics with his series of lectures on the same theme that were eventually published in 2001 in his book, *The Future of Man*. So here we have two philosophers who are able to influence those in power but not be themselves in power! It is our contention that in making the human genome the common heritage of mankind the philosopher should assume the role of 'political catalyst' by influencing those in power without he or she being in power.

Habermas has supported the decision of German legislators to ban several forms of biotechnology that, according to him, 'crossed the line between the 'outer' and 'inner' nature of the human being'.[765] These include pre-natal genetic diagnosis, any research involving the destruction of embryos, therapeutic cloning, 'surrogate motherhood' and medically assisted suicide.[766] The problem with pre-natal genetic diagnosis, for example, is that foetuses possessing some form of genetic disease or some other abnormality will be aborted as they would be considered unworthy of life. Other infants that somehow slip through pre-natal diagnosis will be considered mistakes or rejects that should have never been born![767] Together with pre-natal genetic diagnosis, pre-implantation diagnosis and cloning are new biotechnologies that are bound to transform procreation into manufacture with the fulcrum of human life moved from the family to the laboratory! At the same time Habermas does not exclude the possibility of

---

[763]   Habermas, *The Future of Human Nature*, 2005, p. 23.
[764]   Hans Jonas, *Memoirs*, ed. by Christian Wiese and trans. by Krishna Winston (Waltham, Massachusetts: Brandeis University Press, 2008), p. 212.
[765]   Habermas, *The Future of Human Nature*, 2005, p. 23.
[766]   Ibid.
[767]   Kass, *Life, Liberty and the Defence of Dignity*, p. 130.

using pre-natal genetic diagnosis for therapeutic reasons when, for example, such genetic interventions, carried out preferably on somatic cells, can ameliorate extremely damaging monogenetic diseases.[768] It is important, for Habermas, to draw a line between negative eugenics and enhancing eugenics—the problem is that today it has become very difficult to distinguish between biotechnological intervention for enhancement purposes and clinical treatment for therapeutic purposes. Quoting Hans Jonas, Habermas remarks that,

> the more ruthless the intrusion into the makeup of the human genome becomes, the more inextricably the clinical mode of treatment is assimilated to the biotechnological mode of intervention, blurring the intuitive distinction between the grown and the made, the subjective and the objective—with repercussions reaching as far as the self-reference of the person to her bodily existence.[769]

These are the issues that are raised by biotechnology, that threaten the very essence of our humanness and that contemporary society very often fails to understand. Habermas' philosophical reflections on the question of biotechnology are an echo of Martin Heidegger's thoughts on the issue of technology as it affects the human condition. As explained earlier in this study, the problem with technology for Heidegger does not lie in its uses and applications but rather in man's relation to it. Hans Jonas remarks that,

> Technologically mastered nature now again includes man who (up to now) had, in technology, set himself against it as its master.[770]

This is the crux of the matter and this is why it is the role of the philosopher to be a watchman over the biotechnology debate and why it is vital that the philosopher assumes the role of political catalyst in putting forward the proposition that the patent system be remoulded within a new legal framework that sees the human genome as a common heritage of mankind. It is unfortunate that several critics of Habermas' work have taken his views to be a broad-brush ban on practically all new biotechnologies that have emerged in the past twenty years. The problem with Habermas' critics is that they fail to understand the metaphysical understanding of human nature which, to Habermas, cannot be traded for a new understanding of mankind that is emerging from a predominantly reductionist

---

[768]   Habermas, *The Future of Human Nature*, 2005, pp. 69–70.
[769]   Ibid., p. 47.
[770]   Ibid., pp. 47–48.

interpretation of our human nature.[771] Contrary to what many contemporary intellectuals may believe, the human genome is neither the Book of Life nor the Holy Grail of human nature. It is our contention that the biotechnology debate hasn't even commenced because so far, it has dealt with issues of uses and application of biotechnology without considering the philosophical problems that are presupposed by the essence of biotechnology and which everyone appears to ignore. We believe that Leon Kass managed to capture the significance of what we are trying to say when he spoke of the 'wisdom of repugnance' that makes people use words such as 'offensive, grotesque, revolting, repugnant and repulsive' in response to the suggestion of cloning a human being.[772] Habermas managed to capture the same sentiments when on the question of the 'use' of embryos for research, he wrote:

> If I am not mistaken in my assessment of the debate over the 'use' of embryos for research, or over the conditional creation of embryos, it is disgust at something obscene rather than moral indignation proper that comes to be expressed in our emotional reactions. It is the feeling of vertigo that seizes us when the ground beneath our feet, which we believed to be solid, begins to slip.[773]

Commenting on the way bioethics debates are generally conducted, including the Bundestag, Habermas notes that the value of human life, even in its earliest stages, is not considered to be of paramount importance.[774] On the contrary, it would appear that the destruction of embryos is a small loss compared to the benefits that can be derived from this research, including maintaining a competitive edge on both the academic and industrial level and the procreative right of parents for healthy children and new treatments for genetic disease. But should the human embryo be instrumentalized for the uncertain profits and benefits that can be derived from scientific research?[775]

4.11 The Embryo Question

As stated earlier, Habermas approved the German government's ban on not only pre-natal genetic diagnosis but also on stem cell research that involved the destruction of human embryos and therapeutic cloning. His main concern has been

---

[771]   Elizabeth Fenton, 'Liberal Eugenics and Human Nature: Against Habermas', *Hastings Center Report,* 36:6 (2006), pp. 35–42.

[772]   Kass, *Human Cloning*, p. 17.

[773]   Ibid., p. 39.

[774]   Habermas, *The Future of Human Nature*, 2005, p. 68.

[775]   Ibid., p. 70.

that with pre-natal genetic diagnosis and stem cell research, in particular, the pace was set for the instrumentalization of the human species. As a matter of fact, embryo research has been the subject of intense debate among scientists, politicians and philosophers from the moment James Thomson and his colleagues made public the successful results they had obtained in their attempts to harvest human embryonic stem cells. Four years earlier, Thomson had managed to harvest stem cells from monkey embryos and develop the techniques and appropriate mixture for the monkey cells to live in and replicate for more than a year. The human embryos Thomson used were created as part of the IVF process in a fertility clinic but were not transferred to a woman's uterus for eventual implantation and pregnancy purposes. He also developed the appropriate medium for establishing a stable embryonic stem cell line.[776] There are serious ethical problems with Thomson's method of harvesting human embryonic stem cells because in the process, human embryos are destroyed when they arrive at the blastocyst stage. The reason is that after the fifth day, when the cells of the embryo would have differentiated into those of the trophectoderm[777] and the Inner Cell Mass,[778] the cells of the latter are removed and the blastocyst is destroyed in the process. The researchers' interest lies in the cells of the Inner Cell Mass because these cells have the unique capability of 'making' most of the tissue cells of the human body. They are pluripotent cells because unlike the totipotent zygote that is still undifferentiated and therefore capable of producing all human tissue cells, these Inner Cell Mass cells are unable to create the cells of the trophectoderm.

As explained earlier, the procedure was made the subject of a *Dissident Opinion* by Professor Gunther Virt of the European Group of Ethics who found objection to the granting of patents[779] to processes and products that used mate-

---

[776]   Initially Thomson had no intention of developing the appropriate medium for establishing a stable embryonic stem cell line but he was pushed into doing so because the medium used in IVF clinics could only keep the embryos alive for a maximum of three days when he actually needed at least two more days before he could harvest the stem cells.

[777]   The cells of the trophectoderm become the placenta and other membranes that connect it to the uterus.

[778]   The Inner Cell Mass (ICM) is made up of around thirty cells that they will form the embryo itself.

[779]   Prof. Gunter Virt, 'Dissident Opinion', in *Opinion on the Ethical Aspects of Patenting Inventions Involving Human Stem Cells*, by European Group on Ethics in Science and New Technologies to the European Commission, Opinion Number 16, 7 May 2002.

rial obtained by destroying human embryos. Virt expressed concern at the prospect of patenting human embryonic stem cells and human embryonic stem cell lines that used human embryos as source material! To Virt this was a contradiction in terms and a betrayal of the dignity of the human embryo. When Thomson sought to patent a purified preparation of primate embryonic stem cells, including human embryonic stem cells, the Examining Division of the European Patent Office rejected his application on the grounds that it went against public morality.[780]

After appealing the decision, the patent application passed through both the Technical Board of Appeal and the Enlarged Board of Appeal. The ruling of the Enlarged Board of Appeal was given on 25 November 2008 and it was a reiteration of the decision taken by the Examining Division of 13 July 2004. The ruling was that the WARF/Thomson patent application was to be rejected on the grounds that it fell within the exception to patentability of Article 53(a) and Rule 28(c) of the EPC. However, although the Enlarged Board of Appeal banned the destruction of human embryos, it did not go into the issue of the possible patentability of human stem cells or human stem cell cultures.[781] Accordingly, the decision does not as such prevent the patenting of stem cell inventions that do not involve the use of human embryos. It still remains unclear as to whether human embryonic stem cells that are prepared by methods in which embryos remain viable are patentable or not!

The nature of the human genome encapsulates two separate but interconnected dimensions, that of matter and soul. In our contemporary culture this has come to be understood as the notion that our genome is synonymous with our humanness. For this reason, many philosophers, politicians and scientists have difficulty reconciling the medical benefit that can be eschewed from human embryonic stem cell research with the destruction of human embryos at the blastocyst stage when the cells of the Inner Cell Mass are extricated.

A nod in the right direction was given by the US President, George W. Bush who, in August 2001, put the brakes on embryonic stem cell research when

---

[780] European Patent Office, *Decision of the Enlarged Board of Appeal of 25 November 2008* (Case No. 0002/06). Application No. 96903521. <http://www.bettinger.de/fileadmin/media­pool/downloads/rechtsdatenbank/patent/Urteile/Gooo2_06_en_StemCells.pdf> [accessed on 15 December 2008]

[781] The Enlarged Board of Appeal based its ruling on the relevant provisions of the European Patent Convention (Article 53 (a) and Rule 28 (c) and on the EU Biotechnology Directive (98/44/EC) that was implemented in the European Patent Convention in 1999.

he declared the research to be immoral but allowed research to continue on stem cells already in existence the day he made the speech.[782] President Bush's ban on embryonic stem cell research proved a challenge to many interested researchers to look for alternative sources of stem cells. In fact, after the ban, the National Institutes of Health spent more than $360 million on adult stem cell research for 2002 and 2003 compared with just $35 million on embryonic stem cell research for the same period.

Then in May 2005, the President's Council on Bioethics published a White Paper with four alternative proposals to embryonic stem cell research. The White Paper was not meant to be a collection of four Quick-Start manuals for stem cell research that did not utilize embryos as basic raw material for the research. Rather, it was a poignant statement by some of the leading scientists and bioethicists of American society that the treasure map leading to the magical stem cells had still to be deciphered and that those who saw no other route to these stem cells other than through the destruction of human embryos were blinded by the technological virus that sees, as the ultimate project of modern science, the complete mastery of nature, including human nature. This is the *malaise* of biotechnology that has its origin in the 1970s with the commercialization of academic research. The Huang-Gate fraud of 2005 is a symptom of this *malaise*—in a 2005 paper in *Science* magazine co-authored with Gerald Schatten, Woo Suk Huang laid claim to eleven cloned, patient-specific stem cell lines when in fact there were only two, of which his collaborators took photographs to make them appear to be eleven different stem cell lines.[783]

The road taken by the researchers from the adult stem cell camp led to a significant breakthrough with the work of Shinya Yamanaka from Kyoto University. Yamanaka was an assistant professor doing research on embryonic stem cells when a visit to a friend's fertility clinic changed his career in a way that he had never dreamed possible. Invited by his friend to look through the microscope and to see how a human embryo actually looked like, Yamanaka was struck with awe at the sight of the embryo and realized that it was no different from his two little daughters. That look through the microscope proved to be, for Yamanaka, a life-changing experience that made him turn his back on embryonic stem cell research in order to look for another route to the elusive stem cells. After years of searching and often despair, Yamanaka found the road that

---

[782]   Fox, *Cell of Cells*, p. 20.

[783]   Eve Herold, *Stem Cell Wars: Inside Stories from the Frontlines* (New York: Palgrave Macmillan, 2006), pp. 194–96.

leads to the treasure trove of human tissue regeneration when he succeeded in changing adult skin cells into the equivalent human embryonic stem cells without actually using one single human embryo in the process! The key to Yamanaka's success in procuring stem cells without destroying human embryos was provided by cloning which required that the adult nucleus be reprogrammed by some factors in the egg cell. He succeeded in creating the first 'induced pluripotent stem cells' by inserting four genes, Oct4, Sox2, Klf4 and Myc, into adult human skin cells, inducing the skin cells to revert to the embryonic state.

Yamanaka's procedure was in fact proposal 4 in the White Paper published by the President's Council on Bioethics.[784] The moral advantage of Yamanaka's procedure is that it reaffirms the inviolability of human life across all its stages, from the moment of conception to natural death. The same can be said of another procedure for creating stem cells, listed in the White Paper as Proposal 3 and the brain child of William Hurlburt.[785] Called Altered Nuclear transfer, the procedure involves modifying somatic cell nucleus transfer in such a way that instead of creating a cloned embryo by replacing the nucleus of an oocyte with the nucleus of the somatic cell, the nucleus of the somatic cell is modified before it is transferred to the oocyte thus producing a biological entity that is a source of pluripotent stem cells but not a human embryo.

A 'Thought Experiment' by Markus Grompe of the Oregon Stem Cell Centre explains the general concept behind Altered Nuclear Transfer:

> If you were to introduce messenger RNA for the potent myogenic transcription factor myoD into an oocyte before nuclear transfer, the resulting cell would probably express a muscle phenotype and would, certainly not be an embryo. As the goal of ANT is not to make muscle cells, but pluripotent stem cells, the proposed genetic alterations would ensure that only the inner cell mass, but not trophectoderm lineage, develops after muscle transfer. The differentiation of the embryo into trophectoderm, which gives rise to the placenta, and inner cell mass, which produces the embryo proper, is the first indication that a human organism is present. Conversely, the absence of this step indicates that this cell was not a human embryo.[786]

Both Yamanaka's and Hulburt's techniques for procuring stem cells are free from the ethical concerns that are associated with embryonic stem cells because

---

784 President's Council on Bioethics, *Alternative Sources of Human Pluripotent Stem Cells: A White Paper* (Washington D.C.: May 2005), pp. 50–54.

785 Ibid., pp. 36–50.

786 Markus Grompe, 'Alternative Energy for Embryonic Stem Cell Research', *Nature Reports: Stem Cells* (Published online 11 November 2007 / doi:10.1038/stemcells.2007.100) <http://www.nature.com/stemcells/2007/0710/071011/full/stemcells.2007.100.html> [accessed on 20 January 2008]

they do not entail the destruction of human embryos. Ontologically, the biological entity created by Hurlburt's technique of Altered Nuclear Transfer is different from a human embryo. Both methods are extremely promising for the future and are genuine alternatives to embryonic stem cell research.

The essence of our humanness is to be found in the human genome that represents both our individual and collective identity as a species. The human genome became a major topic of concern within the bioethical field with the launching of the HGP and when the question of whether the human genome should be manipulated began to be raised in public discourse. It is unfortunate that many of the concerns raised by Heidegger on modern technology, Jonas on biotechnological engineering and Gadamer on issues of medical ethics are very often absent from this public debate. With the exception of Jurgen Habermas, contemporary philosophers have shunned from becoming directly involved in the public debate on biotechnology and the human genome.

If in the negotiations that led to the Law of the Sea the work of Hugo Grotius was a constant work of reference for the negotiators, in the negotiations that must lead to a Law of the Human Genome, the works of Arvid Pardo, Martin Heidegger, Hans Jonas, Hans-Georg Gadamer and Jurgen Habermas must be the rich philosophical sources from which the political negotiators of the human genome as common heritage of mankind must draw inspiration. The reason is because the question of making the human genome the common heritage of mankind is first and foremost a philosophical issue that must make compassionate humanism understand, in the interests of all mankind, that the time has come to make the human genome, as a common heritage of mankind, a legal norm of international law.

Conclusions

The human genome and the concept of common heritage of mankind were chosen as subjects of my thesis because the commercialization of the genome has
not reduced its pace and every effort is being made, from the world of politics
and science, to discredit those who are trying to restore some sense of dignity to
the human genome in the interests of humanity. The concept of common heritage of mankind can be the ideal jacket to fit the human genome as the embodiment of our true humanness that defies reductionism to physico-chemical quan-
tification.

The timeline of the human genome as common heritage of mankind is
marked by significant political decisions that have required courage and determination from individuals and groups that have refused to compromise on the
issue of the inviolability of human life. Through the course of our study we have
tried to explain that there is more to biotechnology than simply finding ways
and means for saving life by avoiding death and suffering. Leon Kass, ex-Chair-
man of the President's Council on Bioethics, expressed the sentiments of many
concerned individuals, including ourselves, when he commented that, 'en-
chanted and enslaved by the glamour of technology we have lost our awe and
wonder before the deep mysteries of nature and life'.[787] And what is the human
genome if not the embodiment of the deep mysteries of our humanness!

Arvid Pardo gave us the conceptual tool that we need to preserve the dignity of our genome when he put to the General Assembly of the United Nations
his proposal to make the deep seabed the common heritage of mankind.[788] Pardo
introduced into the political arena an apparently new regime of international
management that has been the subject of heated debate since its inception.
Pardo's concept of common heritage of mankind was primarily a philosophical
concept in that it was not meant to merely introduce another form of property
management but rather to change peoples' minds and hearts in the interests of
all humanity by establishing an international authority that would manage the
deep seabed for and on behalf of all mankind. A fundamental notion of the Pardosian concept of common heritage of mankind that is lacking in most scholarly

---

[787] Kass, 'Wisdom of Repugnance', p. 10.
[788] Universal Declaration on the Human Genome and Human Rights, adopted by the General Conference of UNESCO at its 29th Session on 11 November 1997 and adopted by the United
Nations General Assembly at its 53rd Session on 9 December 1998 with Resolution 53/152.

essays on the subject concerns the possibility, under certain circumstances, of 'refraining' from using the common heritage in the interests of all mankind. This is the fundamentally innovative notion of management that Pardo sought to make the international community comprehend in the many debates that followed his initial address to the General Assembly. As has been demonstrated in this study, in the twilight years of his life, Pardo saw the concept of common heritage of mankind as originally proposed and intended by him, become nothing more than a political slogan in the hands of several leaders of the most industrialized countries including the United States, who had no intention of relinquishing their property rights.

The concept of common heritage of mankind resurfaced in 1997 when the General Conference of UNESCO declared that the human genome was, 'in a symbolic sense, the heritage of humanity'.[789] The Declaration was soon followed by the launching of the HGP with the goal of identifying the 3 billion or so nucleotides that made up the human genome. As explained in our study, there never was the political will to manage the HGP along the lines of Arvid Pardo's concept of common heritage of mankind. The US and UK leaders paid lip service to the concept of common heritage of mankind when, in their Joint Statement, they declared that the human genome should remain in the public domain. [790] The race to complete the HGP became a race to patent as much of it as possible with the ensuing anti-commons effect that paralysed biomedical research and delayed providing people with better medical care.

When Arvid Pardo addressed the UN General Assembly and put forward the notion that the deep seabed be made the common heritage of mankind, he spoke of the sense of urgency that impelled him to call on the member states of the UN to take immediate action so as to put a halt to the unilateral exploitation of the deep seabed resources by the industrialized nations that had the finances and the technology to do so.[791] The same sense of urgency to take immediate action to give true credence to the UNESCO Declaration that the human genome be made the common heritage of mankind is felt today when, from all quarters, fundamental boundaries that up to twenty-five years ago universally defined our

---

[789]   Ibid.

[790]   Rimmer, *Intellectual Property and Biotechnology*, p. 141.

[791]   Address by Arvid Pardo to the 22nd session of the General Assembly of the United Nations (1967), Official records of the General Assembly, 22nd Session, Agenda item 92, Document A/6695.

humanness are being obfuscated by technological change and risk being lost to posterity.

The purpose of this study has been to put the human genome at the centre of human concern. As stated earlier, the concept of common heritage of mankind as originally proposed by Arvid Pardo to the UN General Assembly is the ideal jacket that fits the human genome today more than ever when the human genome has fallen victim to the demands of modern technology and invisible hand mechanisms that are typical of the instrumental reasoning that dominates modern society.

The concept of common heritage of mankind can constitute the *nexus* between biotechnology and the human genome. In this sense it is the concept of common heritage of mankind that can restore meaning and significance to the human genome as the embodiment of our humanity! This will entail re-ordering our relation to biotechnology in the Heideggerian ideal of tapping the 'redemptive quality' inherent in it and moving from a passive submission to biotechnology to a critical and questioning relationship to biotechnology that is continually making incursions into our lives. Heidegger's discussion of technology is not centred on the ethical legitimacy of particular technologies but on the thinking that lies behind the whole domain of technology. It is Martin Heidegger's reflections on technology combined with the work of other philosophers who have reflected on both technology and biotechnology that can lead us to higher forms of existence that are essentially related to how we perceive and relate to the human genome.

Fundamentally, the application of the concept of common heritage of mankind to the human genome entails duties of obligation that are concomitant with assuming the responsible stewardship of the human genome. But with Arvid Pardo's notion of the common heritage of mankind as proposed to the UN General Assembly, the notion of stewardship does not remain a vague moral obligation but, on the contrary, the idea of international management for and on behalf of all mankind provides a political model of how this can be achieved. With the human genome this political model can be launched by the establishment of the International Human Genome Authority as proposed earlier in our study. But other initiatives must and can be taken in the immediate future with firm determination if the concept of common heritage of mankind is not to suffer the same fate it met with UNCLOS III and the Law of the Sea.

One such bold initiative was taken by two US Congressman, Xavier Becerra and Dave Weldon, in 2007, when they introduced the *Genomic Research and Accessibility Act* to put an end to the patenting of any and all portions of the human genome. This bill is intended to amend the Patent Act of 1952 by prohibiting the patenting of genetic material. According to Representative Becerra, once the bill becomes law, in less than twenty years we will have a patent-free genome! In Representative Becerra's words,

One-fifth of the blueprint that makes up you...me...and my children...your children...all...of us...is owned by someone else...And we have absolutely no say in what those entities do with our genes. This cannot be what Watson and Crick intended.

We seek simply to fix a regulatory mistake. Genes are a product of nature; they were not created by man, but instead are the very blueprint that creates man, and thus, are not patentable. Gene patenting would be the analogous equivalent to patenting water, air, birds or diamonds.

Enacting the Genomic Research and Accessibility Act does not hamper invention, indeed, it encourages it. The proliferation of scientific prowess, medical innovation and economic advancement will all occur if the study of genes is allowed to happen unabated. Incredible manifestations of intellectual property will result: medicines, machines, processes—most deserving of recognition, some potentially life-saving, and all worthy of a patent.[792]

Initiatives must be taken from all quarters to change the concept of common heritage of mankind from a philosophical concept grounded in natural law to a legal principle of international law. On the international level, Malta could take the initiative to recommend to the UNESCO General Conference to explain to the member states the reasons why the human genome was only referred to as 'in a symbolic sense, the heritage of humanity'. As has been explained earlier, the reason was to avoid any reductionist interpretations of the human genome but unfortunately the expression, 'in a symbolic sense', proved to be both vague and ambiguous. The other alternative would be for Malta to recommend to the UNESCO General Conference that Article 1 of the Declaration on the Human Genome and Human Rights should no longer include the qualification 'in a symbolic sense' when stating that the human genome is the common heritage of humanity. The wording of the Article, as it stands, is not conducive to making the human genome, as common heritage of mankind, a legal principle of international law. Malta should also consider using the UN General Assembly as a

---

[792]   Rimmer, *Intellectual Property and Biotechnology*, pp. 156–57.

platform to propose an international debate on applying the principle of non-patentability to the human genome.

Few speeches heard at the UN General Assembly generated as much activity as did Arvid Pardo's speech of 1 November 1967. First, an Ad-hoc Committee was formed to study Pardo's proposal and make recommendations to the General Assembly; second, the Committee was reconstituted as a Permanent Committee on the Peaceful Uses of the Seabed and Ocean Floor Beyond the Limits of National Jurisdiction[793]; third, in 1969, two other resolutions were passed, namely the Moratorium Resolution[794] and the Resolution on Marine Space[795] with which the UN General Assembly expressed its support for the International Decade of Ocean Exploration (1971–1980) proposed by the US; fourth, the Soviet Union and the US submitted proposals for the demilitarization of the seabed which in 1971 led to the Treaty on the Prohibition of the Emplacement of Nuclear Weapons and Other Weapons of Mass Destruction on the Sea-Bed and Ocean Floor and in the Subsoil Thereof[796]; fifth, the UN General Assembly adopted a Declaration of Principles Governing the Seabed and the Ocean Floor, and the Subsoil Thereof, beyond the Limits of National Jurisdiction[797]; sixth, in 1970 the UN General Assembly decided to convene in 1973 a Conference on the Law of the Sea[798]. Malta can once again be the catalyst that sets the wheels in motion for the world community to change its stance vis-à-vis the human genome and make the human genome, as a common heritage of mankind, a legal principle of international law.

Throughout the course of this thesis, two themes have been constantly in my mind and these are (i) the urgent need to put the human genome on the political agenda of the world community and (ii) to create, among the world community, an awareness of the dangers posed by technology, in particular biotechnology, to our humanness. The questions posed by Heidegger, the concerns about illness and health of Gadamer, the reflections of Habermas on the future of man, the 'heuristics of fear' of Hans Jonas, the ethical concerns of Paul Ramsey and the wise reflections on modern society of Leon Kass, among others, cannot be ignored.

---

[793] UNGA Resolution 2467A (XXIII).
[794] UNGA Resolution 2574D (XXIV).
[795] UNGA Resolution 2560 (XXIV).
[796] Seabed Treaty that entered into force on 18 May 1972.
[797] UNGA Resolution 2749 (XXV).
[798] UNGA Resolution 2750 (XXV).

I hope to have succeeded in exploring the issue of biotechnology from a philosophical perspective together with the notion of common heritage of mankind as applied to the human genome to demonstrate that it is precisely the concept of common heritage of mankind that can save the human genome which is the embodiment of our humanness, from the dehumanizing effect of biotechnology. It will not be any easy task just as it was not an easy task for Arvid Pardo to make the deep seabed a common heritage of mankind. But the hold of the patent system on human genomic research must not be allowed to prevail. Every man, woman and child who dies because he or she is denied a vital drug that is not manufactured by a pharmaceutical company because it is not profitable to do so, is a victim of a patenting system that was originally intended to encourage research and innovation but is now used to restrain biomedical research for economic profit. But here we are talking about research that uses as resource material **my genome** and **your genome** and not some biological entity that is outside of ourselves. It follows that human genomic research should only be used and never owned by any individual or private and public companies. Any benefit derived from this research should also be shared among all mankind considering the essential connection that exists between our genome and our humanity. Since this research has as its resource material our human genome that resides in our universal human nature, it should only be used for exclusively peaceful purposes for and on behalf of all mankind. Considering the universal nature of the human genome, the management of the human genome by an international representation of all mankind appears to be the most idoneous arrangement! Put differently, the human genome has always belonged to the common heritage of mankind and today, more than in the past, this presents itself as a moral and political obligation to assume the responsible stewardship of the human genome.

Bibliography

Council of Europe

Additional Protocol to the Convention on Human Rights and Biomedicine Concerning Biomedical Research, Strasbourg, 25 January 2005, CETS n. 195.

Additional Protocol to the Convention on Human Rights and Biomedicine Concerning Transplantation of Organs and Tissues of Human Origin, Strasbourg, 24 January 2002, CETS n. 186.

Additional Protocol to the Convention for the Protection of Human Rights and Dignity of the Human Being with regard to the Application of Biology and Medicine on the Prohibition of Cloning Human Beings, Paris, 12 January 1998, CETS n. 168.

Convention for the Protection of Human Rights and Dignity of the Human Being with Regard to the Application of Biology and Medicine: Convention on Human Rights and Biomedicine, Oviedo, 4 April 1997, CETS n. 164.

Parliamentary Assembly of the Council of Europe Recommendation 1468 (2000) on Biotechnologies.

Parliamentary Assembly of the Council of Europe Recommendation 1425 (1999) on Biotechnology and Intellectual Property, para. 8.

Parliamentary Assembly of the Council of Europe Recommendation 1512 (2001) on the Protection of the Human Genome.

European Union

Case C – 377/98, Kingdom of the *Netherlands* v. *European Parliament and Council of the European Union*, Judgment of the Full Court of 9 October 2001. [2001] ECR 1-07079.

Directive 96/9/EC of the European Parliament and of the Council of 11 March 1996 on the Legal Protection of Databases. OJL 77, 27 March 1996.

Directive 98/44/EC of the European Parliament and of the Council of 6 July 1998 on the Legal Protection of Biotechnological Inventions. OJL 213, 30 July 1998.

European Group on Ethics in Science and New Technologies to the European Commission, *Opinion on the Ethical Aspects of Patenting Inventions Involving Human Stem Cells*, Opinion Number 16, 7 May 2002.

Opinion of the Economic and Social Committee on the 'Proposal for a European Parliament and Council Directive on the Legal Protection of Biotechnological Inventions'. OJ, C295 of 7 October 1996.

European Patent Office

Convention on the Grant of European Patents (European Patent Convention), 12th Ed., (Munich: European Patent Office, 2006).

Decision of the Enlarged Board of Appeal for the Non-Patentability of Inventions Involving the Use and Destruction of Human Embryos. (25 November 2008).

European Patent Convention (EPC 1973). <http://www.epo.org/patents/law/legal-texts /html/epc/1973/e/ma1.html> [accessed on 12 June 2007]

European Patent Office. <http://www.epo/org> [accessed on 12 June 2007]

United Nations

Agreement Governing the Activities of States on the Moon and Other Celestial Bodies, adopted by the General Assembly of the United Nations at its 34th Session on 14 December 1979. UNGA Res. 34/68.

Agreement Relating to the Implementation of Part XI of the United Nations Convention on the Law of the Sea (10 December 1982) of 28 July 1994. UNGA Res. 48/263.

Charter of the United Nations, signed in San Francisco on 26 June 1945, at the conclusion of the United Nations Conference on International Organization.

Declaration on the Establishment of a New Economic Order, adopted by the General Assembly of the United Nations at its Sixth Special Session on 1 May 1974. UN Doc. A/9556.

Declaration on Human Cloning, adopted by the General Assembly of the United Nations at its 59th Session on 8 March 2005. UNGA Res. 59/280.

Declaration of the Principles Governing the Seabed and the Ocean Floor, and the Subsoil Thereof, beyond the Limits of National Jurisdiction, adopted by the General Assembly of the United Nations at its 25th Session on 17 December 1970. UNGA Res. 2749 (XXV).

Declaration of the United Nations Conference on the Human Environment, proclaimed in Stockholm on 16 June 1972.

Rio Declaration on Environment and Development, proclaimed at the conclusion of the United Nations Conference on Environment and Development in Rio de Janeiro on 14 June 1992.

Treaty on Principles Governing the Activities of States in the Exploration and Use of Outer Space, including the Moon and Other Celestial Bodies, adopted by the General Assembly of the United Nations at its 21st Session on 19 December 1966. UNGA Res. 2222 (XXI).

United Nations 1979 Agreement Governing the Activities of States on the Moon and Other Celestial Bodies, adopted by the General Assembly of the United Nations at its 34th Session on 5 December 1979. UNGA Resolution 34/68.

United Nations Convention on the Law of the Sea (UNCLOS), Montego Bay, 10 December 1982.

UNGA Res 2749 (XXV) on the Declaration of Principles Governing the Seabed and the Ocean Floor, and the Subsoil Thereof, beyond the Limits of National Jurisdiction, adopted by the General Assembly of the United Nations at its 25th Session on 17 December 1970.

UNGA Res. 53/152 on The Human Genome and Human Rights, adopted by the United Nations General Assembly at its 53rd Session on 9 December 1998.

UNGA Res. 43/53 on the Protection of Global Climate for Present and Future Generations of Mankind, adopted on 6 December 1988.

UNGA Res 2574 (XXIII) on the Question of the Reservation for Exclusively Peaceful Purposes of the Seabed and Ocean Floor, and the Subsoil Thereof, Underlying the High Seas beyond the Limits of National Jurisdiction, and the Use of Their Resources in the Interests of Mankind, adopted by the General Assembly of the United Nations at its 24th Session on 15 December 1969.

Universal Declaration of Human Rights, adopted by the General Assembly of the United Nations at its 3rd Session on 10 December 1948. UNGA Res. 217 A (III).

World Charter for Nature, adopted by the General Assembly of the United Nations at its 37th Session on 28 October 1982. UNGA Res. 37/7.

UNESCO

Convention for the Protection of Cultural Property in the Event of Armed Conflict, adopted at The Hague (Netherlands) on 14 May 1954.

Convention Concerning the Protection of the World Cultural and Natural Heritage, adopted by the General Conference of UNESCO at its 17th Session on 16 November 1972.

Declaration of the Principles of International Cultural Co-operation, adopted by the General Conference of UNESCO at its 14th Session on 4 November 1966.

International Declaration on Human Genetic Data, adopted by the General Conference of UNESCO at its 32nd Session on 16 October 2003.

Universal Declaration on the Human Genome and Human Rights, adopted by the General Conference of UNESCO at its 29th Session on 11 November 1997.

USPTO

Peoples Business Commission, Appellate Brief of Peoples' Business Commission as Amici Curiae in Support of the Petitioner in 'Diamond v Chakrabarty', WL 2005 (13 December 1979).

United States Patent and Trademark Office. <http://www.uspto.gov/> [accessed on 12 June 2007]

United States Patent and Trademark Office, *General Information Concerning Patents* (Washington D.C.: Patent and Trademark Office, 1999).

United States Patent and Trademark Office, 2106 Patent Subject Matter Eligibility [R-6] 2100 Patentability (26 October 2005). <http://www.gov/web/offices/pac/mpep/doc uments/2100_2106htm> [accessed on 18 April 2006]

United States Patent and Trademark Office (1999), 'Revised Interim Utility Examination Guidelines', Federal Register, vol.64 no. 244. <http://www.uspto.gov/web/offi ces/com/sol/notices/utilexmguide.pdf> [accessed on 18 April 2005]

United States Patent and Trademark Office (2001), Utility Examination Guidelines', Federal Register, vol. 66. no. 4. <http://www.uspto.gov/web/offices/com/sol/no-tices/utilexmguide.pdf> [accessed on 14 March 2005]

Encyclicals

Pope John XXIII – Pacem in Terris, 1963. <http://www.vatican.va/holy_father/john _xxiii/encyclicals/documents/hf_j-xxiii_enc_11041963_pacem_en.html> [accessed on 15 September 2007]

Pope Paul VI – De Populorum Progressio, 1967. <http://www.vatican.va/holy_father/pa ul_vi/encyclicals/documents/hf_p-vi_enc_26031967_populorum_en.html> [accessed on 15 September 2007]

Pope Pius XI, Quaragesimo Anno, 1931. <http://www.vatican.va/holy_father/piu s_xi/encyclicals/documents/hf_p-xi_enc_19310515_quadragesimo-anno_en.html> [accessed on 15 September 2007]

International Legislation

Antarctic Treaty (1959). Antarctic Connection. <http://www.antarcticconnection.com/a ntarctic/treaty/index.shtml> [accessed on 20 January 2006]

International Organizations

Statement on Benefit-Sharing by the HUGO Ethics Committee, released on 9 April 2000.

World Medical Association Declaration of Helsinki: Ethical Principles for Medical Research Involving Human Subjects, adopted by the 18th World Medical Association and amended by the 52nd WMA General Assembly, Edinburgh, Scotland, October 2000.

National Legislation

Bayh-Dole Act (The Patent and Trademark Law Amendments Act), enacted into law and passed by the United States Congress on 12 December 1980. P.L. 96-517.

Law on the Exploration and Exploitation of the Mineral Resources of the Deep Seabed 1985, 24 ILM 983 (1985) Italy.

Deep Seabed Hard Minerals Resources Act 1980 (USA).

Law on the Exploration and Exploitation of the Mineral Resources of the Deep Seabed 1985 (Italy).

Law on Interim Measures for Deep Seabed Mining 1983 (Japan).

Edict on Provisional Measures to Regulate Soviet Enterprises for the Exploration and Exploitation of Mineral Resources 1982 (USSR).

Deep Sea Mining (Temporary Provisions) Act 1981 (UK).

Act of Interim Regulation of Deep Seabed Mining 1982 (Federal Republic of Germany).

Books and Articles

Abdy, John Thomas and Bryan Walker, *The Institutes of Justinian* (Cambridge: Cambridge University Press, 1876).

Agius, Emmanuel, 'Patenting Life: Our Responsibilities to Present and Future Generations', in *Germ-Line Intervention and our Responsibilities to Future Generations*, ed. by Emmanuel Agius and Salvino Busuttil (Dordrecht: Kluwer Academic Publishers, 1998).

Agius, Emmanuel and Lionel Chircop, Caring for Future Generations: Jewish, Christian and Islamic Perspectives (Westport, Conn: Praeger, 1998).

Anand, Ram Prakash, Legal Regime of the Deep Sea-Bed and the Developing Countries (Delhi: Thompson Press, 1975).

Andorno, Roberto, 'Human Dignity and the UNESCO Declaration on the Human Genome' in *Ethics, Law and Society*, ed. by Jennifer Gunning and Soren Holm (Aldershot: Ashgate, 2005).

Andrews, Lori, 'Genes and Patent Policy: Rethinking Intellectual Property Rights', *Nature Reviews Genetics*, 3 (2002), 803–08.

Aquinas, St. Thomas, *Summa Theologiae: Injustice*, ed./trans. by Marcus Lefebure O.P., 60 vols (London: Blackfriars, 1975), XXXVIII.

- - - *Summa Theologiae: Law and Political Theory*, ed. /trans. by Thomas Gilby O.P., 60 vols (London: Blackfriars, 1975), XXVIII.

- - - *Summa Theologiae: The Trinity*, ed. / trans. by Timothy Sutton, 60 vols (London: Blackfriars, 1975), VI.

- - - *Summa Theologiae: Sin*, ed. /trans. by John Fearon O.P., 60 vols (London: Blackfriars, 1975), XXV.

Aristotle, *The Metaphysics*, trans. by Hugh Lawson-Tancred (London: Penguin Books, 2004).

- - - 'On the Soul', in *The Complete Works of Aristotle*, ed. by Jonathan Barnes, 2 vols (Princetown; Princetown University Press, 1995).

- - - *Physics*, trans. by Robin Waterfield (Oxford: Oxford University Press, 1999).

- - - 'Poetics', in *The Complete Works of Aristotle*, ed. by Jonathan Barnes, 2 vols (Princetown: Princetown University Press, 1984).

Barard Judith, *The Ethics of Star Trek* (New York: Perennial, 2001).

Barkenbus, Jack, *Deep Seabed Resources: Politics and Technology* (New York: Free Press, 1979).

Baslar, Kemal, The Concept of the Common Heritage of Mankind in International Law (The Hague: Martinus Nijhoff Publishers, 1998).

Bearley, Helen, The Patentability of Stem Cells, 2008. <http://www.elkfife.com/view_article.php?id=70> [accessed on 2 January 2009]

Beck, P.J., 'The United Nations and Antarctica, 2005: The End of the "Question of Antarctica"?', *Polar Record*, 42:3 (2006), 217–27.

Bederman, David J., *Counterintuiting Countermeasures*, quoted in Peter S. Prows, *Tough Love: The Dramatic Birth and Looming Demise of UNCLOS Property Law*, New York University Public Law and Legal Theory Working Papers, Paper 30 (2006). < http://ssrn.com/abstract=918458> [accessed 15 June 2008]

Benowitz, Steve, 'French Challenge to BRCA1 Patent Underlies European Discomfort', *Journal of National Cancer Institute*, 94 (2002), 80–81.

Biermann, F., 'Saving the Atmosphere: International Law, Developing Countries and Air Pollution', *European Journal of International Law*, 10:3 (1999), 549–82.

Bloch, Ernest, *Natural Law and Human Dignity*, quoted in Esther D. Reed, 'Property Rights, Genes and Common Good', *Journal of Religious Ethics*, 34:1 (2006), 41–67.

Boczek, Boleslaw, *Ideology and the Law of the Sea: The Challenge of the New International Economic Order*, quoted in Edward Guntrip, 'The Common Heritage of Mankind: An Adequate Regime for Managing the Deep Seabed', *Melbourne Journal of International Law*, 4:2 (2003). <http://www.mjil.law.unimelb.edu.au/iss ues/archive/2003(2)/02Guntrip.pdf> [accessed on 10 May 2006]

Bollier, David, Silent Thief: The Private Plunder of Our Common Wealth (New York: Routledge, 2003).

Bovenberg, Jasper A., Inalienably Yours? The New Case for an Inalienable Property Right in Human Biological Material: Empowerment of Sample Donors or a Recipe for a Tragic Anti-Commons? (2004) 1:4 SCRIPT-ed 545. <http://www.law.ed.ac.u k/ahrb/script-ed/issue4/bovenberg.asp> [accessed on 20 January 2007]

Bovenberg, Jasper A., *Property Rights in Blood, Genes and Data: Naturally Yours?* (Leiden: Martinus Nijhoff Publishers, 2006).

Boyle, Joseph, 'Natural Law, Ownership and the World's Natural Resources', in *Thomas Aquinas*, ed. by John Inglis (Aldershot: Ashgate, 2006).

Buber, Martin, *I and Thou*, trans. by Ronald Gregor Smith (Edinburgh: T&TClark, 1999).

Buckle, Stephen, 'Natural Law', in *A Companion to Ethics*, ed. by Peter Singer (Oxford: Blackwell Publishers, 1993).

Bull, Hedley, 'The Importance of Grotius in the Study of International Relations' in *Hugo Grotius and International Relations*, ed. by Benedict Kingsbury, Hedley Bull and Adam Roberts (Oxford: Clarendon Press, 1990).

Chakrabarty, A.M., 'Patenting Life Forms: Yesterday, Today and Tomorrow', in *Perspectives on Properties of the Human Genome Project*, ed. by F. Scott Kieff and John M. Olin (Amsterdam: Elsevier Academic Press, 2003).

Check, Erika, 'Canada Stops Harvard's Oncomouse in its Tracks', *Nature*, 420 (12 December 2002), 593.

Churchill, R.R. and A.V. Lowe, *The Law of the Sea* (Manchester: Manchester University Press, 1999).

Clinton, Bill and Tony Blair, Joint Statement by President William Clinton and Prime Minister Tony Blair of the United Kingdom (14 March 2000). <http://www.ip-mall.info/hosted_resources/ippresdocs/ippd_44.htm, 14 March> [accessed on 20 March 2006]

Cocca, A.A., *The Law of Mankind: Ius Inter Gentes Again*, quoted in Kemal Baslar, *The Concept of Common Heritage of Mankind in International Law* (The Hague: Matinus Nijhoff Publishers, 1998).

Cohen, Eric, *In the Shadow of Progress: Being Human in the Age of Technology* (New York: Encounter Books, 2008).

Committee for the Study of Ethical Aspects of Human Reproduction for the International Federation of Gynecology and Obstetrics, *Patenting of Human Genes* 1997. <http://www.figo.org/> [accessed on 20 January 2006]

Condella, Craig A., Overcoming the Destining of Technological Being. Symposium: Humanity's Place in the Cosmos (6 November 2001). <http://www.fordham.edu/philo sophy/fps/symposia/2001fall/condella.htm> [accessed on 28 November 2008]

Cotterrell, Roger, *The Politics of Jurisprudence* (London: Butterworths, 1989).

Crick, Francis, *Of Molecules and Men* (New York: Prometheus Books, 2004).

Dallmayr, Fred, 'The Enigma of Health: Hans-Georg Gadamer at 100', *The Review of Politics*, 62 (2000), 327–50.

Darwin, Charles, *The Origin of Species: By Means of Natural Selection* (Middlesex: Senate, 1998).

Dawkins, Richard, 'A Reply to Poole', *Science & Christian Belief*, 7:1, No. 1 (1995), 45–50.

- - - *The Blind Watchmaker: Why the Evidence of Evolution Reveals a Universe Without Design*, 2nd edn (New York: W.W. Norton & Company, 1996).

- - - *The Selfish Gene,* 30th Anniversary edn (Oxford: Oxford University Press, 2006).

De Chardin, Teilhard, *Building the Earth* (London: Geoffrey Chapman, 1965).

- - - *The Divine Milieu* (New York: Perennial, 2001).

- - - *The Future of Man,* trans. by Norman Denny (New York: Doubleday, 2004).

- - - *The Phenomenon of Man*, trans. by Bernard Hall (New York: Harper & Row Publishers, 1975).

- - - *The Vision of the Past*, trans. by J.M. Cohen (London: Collins 1966).

Demaine, I.J. and A.X. Fellmeth, 'Reinventing the Double Helix: A Novel and Nonobvious Reconceptualization of the Biotechnology Patent', *Standard Law Review*, 55 (2002), 303–462.

Dennett, Daniel C., *Darwin's Dangerous Idea: Evolution and the Meanings of Life* (New York: Simon & Schuster, 1996).

Dias, W.P.S., 'Heidegger's Relevance for Engineering: Questioning Technology', *Science and Engineering Ethics*, 9:3 (2003), 389–96.

Eberl, Jason T., *Thomistic Principles and Bioethics* (London: Routledge, 2006).

Eight Meeting of the Legal Commission of the International Bioethics Committee' (Paris, 16–17 December 1996), in *Birth of the Universal Declaration of the Human Genome and Human Rights* (Paris: UNESCO, 1999).

Eisenberg, Rebecca, 'How Can You Patent Genes?', in *Who Owns Life?*, ed. by David Magnus, Arthur Caplan and Glenn McGee (New York: Prometheus Books, 2002).

Eisenberg, Rebecca, 'Re-Examining the Role of Patents in Appropriating the Value of DNA Sequences', *Emory Law Journal* 49 (2000), 783–800.

Ellul, Jacques, *The Technological Society*, trans. by John Wilkinson (New York: Vintage Books, 1964).

Fenton, Elizabeth, 'Liberal Eugenics and Human Nature: Against Habermas', *Hastings Center Report,* 36:6 (2006), 35–42.

Filibeck, Giorgio, 'Protecting Human Genome is the Responsibility of all Humanity: Observations on the Human Genome Declaration recently adopted by the General Conference of UNESCO', *L'Osservatore Romano,* 11 February 1998.

Foot, Philippa, *Natural Goodness* (Oxford: Oxford University Press, 2001).

'Fourth Meeting of the Legal Commission of the IBC' (Paris, 27 April 1994), in *Birth of the Universal Declaration of the Human Genome and Human Rights* (Paris: UNESCO, 1999).

Fox, Cynthia, *Cell of Cells: The Global Race to Capture and Control Stem Cell* (New York: W.W. Norton & Company, 2007).

Francioni, Francesco, 'International Law for Biotechnology: Basic Principles', in *Biotechnology and International Law,* ed. by Francesco Francioni and Tullio Scovazzi (Oxford: Hart Publishing, 2006).

Frankl, V.E., 'Reductionism and Nihilism', in *Beyond Reductionism: New Perspectives in the Life Sciences,* ed. by A. Koestler and J.R. Smythies (London: Hutchinson, 1969).

Frohriep Pestalozi, Deborah, *The Case of Anticommons in Biomedical Research* (MAS_IP Diploma Papers & Research Reports), Module 115 'US-Patents' Paper 3 (2006).

Gadamer, Hans-Georg, *The Enigma of Health: The Art of Healing in a Scientific Age* (California: Stanford University Press, 1996).

Garreau, Joel, *Radical Evolution: The Promise and Peril of Enhancing our Minds, Our Bodies—and What it Means to be Human* (New York: Doubleday, 2004).

Global Report, Center for War/Peace Studies 56 (1999/2000). <http://www.cwps.org/old/global56.htm> [accessed on 20 June 2007]

Gold, Richard E. and Timothy Caulfield, 'The Moral Tollbooth: A Method that Makes Use of the Patent System to Address Ethical Concerns in Biotechnology', *Lancet,* 359 (2002), 2268–70.

Goldman, Brian, 'HER2 Testing: The Patent "Genee" Is Out of the Bottle', *Canadian Medical Association Journal,* 176 (2007), 1443–44.

Gould, Stephen J., *I Have Landed: The End of a Beginning in Natural History* (New York: Harmony Books, 2002).

Green, Ronald M., *Babies by Design: The Ethics of Genetic Choice* (New Haven: Yale University Press, 2007).

Grene, Marjorie, 'The Faith of Darwinism', in *The Knower and the Known* (New York: Basic Books, 1966).

- - - 'Reducibility: Another Side Issue?', in *Interpretations of Life and Mind: Essays around the Problem of Reduction*, ed. by Marjorie Grene (London: Routledge and K. Paul, 1971).

- - - 'Time and Teleology', in *The Knower and the Known*, ed. by Marjorie Grene (New York: Basic Books, 1966).

Grisez, Germain G., *Abortion: The Myths, the Realities and the Arguments* (New York: Corpus Books, 1970).

Grompe, Markus, Alternative Energy for Embryonic Stem Cell Research, Nature Reports: Stem Cells (Published online 11 November 2007 / doi:10.1038/stemcells.2007.100). <http://www.nature.com/stemcells/2007/0710/071011/full/stemcells.2007.100.html 11 October 2007> [accessed on 20 January 2008]

Gros Espiell, Hector, *Genese de la Declaration Universelle sur le Genome Humain et les Droits de l'Homme* (Paris: UNESCO, 1999).

- - - 'Project of an International Instrument for the Protection of the Human Genome' (12 September 1994), pp. 41–48, in *Birth of the Universal Declaration on the Human Genome and Human Rights*, Observation 4 (Paris: UNESCO, 1999).

Grotius, Hugo, *Freedom of the Seas: The Right of the Dutch to Take Part in the East Indian Trade*, trans. by Ralph Van Deman Magoffin (New York: Oxford University Press, 1916). <http://www.oll.libertyfund.org/EBOOKS/Grotius_0049.pdf> [accessed on 22 August 2006]

- - - *On the Law of War and Peace*, trans. by A.C. Campbell (London 1814). <http://www.constitution.org/gro/djbp.htm> [accessed on 22 August 2006]

- - - *The Rights of War and Peace*, trans. by A.C. Campbell (New York: M. Walter Dunne, 1901). <http://oll.libertyfund.org/?option=com_staticxt&staticfile=show.php%3Ftitle=553&chapter=90754&layout=html&Itemid=27> [accessed on 20 February 2006]

Guntrip, Edward, 'The Common Heritage of Mankind: An Adequate Regime for Managing the Deep Seabed', *Melbourne Journal of International Law*, 4:2 (2003). <http://www.mjil.law.unimelb.edu.au/issues/archive/2003(2)/02Guntrip.pdf> [accessed on 10 April 2007]

Habermas, Jurgen, *The Future of Human Nature* (Cambridge: Polity Press, 2003).

Hamid, Abdul Wahid, *Islam: The Natural Way*, quoted in Kemal Baslar, *The Concept of Common Heritage of Mankind in International Law* (The Hague: Martinus Nijhoff Publishers, 1998).

Hardin, Garrett, 'The Tragedy of the Commons', *Science* 162 (1968), 1243–48.

Harmon, Shawn, 'The Significance of UNESCO's Universal Declaration on the Human Genome & Human Rights', (2005) 2:1 *SCRIPTed* 20. <http://www.law.ed.ac.u k/ahrc/script-ed/vol2-1/harmon.asp> [accessed on 30 May 2006]

Heidegger, Martin, 'Building Dwelling Thinking', in *Basic Writings* (London: Routledge, 2007).

- - - *Contributions to Philosophy (From Enowning)*, trans. by Parvis Emad Emad and Kenneth Maly (Bloomington, Indiana: Indiana University Press, 1999).

- - - 'The Question Concerning Technology', in *Basic Writings*, ed. by David Farrell Krell (London: Routledge,1978).

- - - 'The Thing', in *Poetry, Language, Thought*, trans. by A. Hofstader (New York: Harper and Row, 1971).

Heller Michael A. and Rebecca S. Eisenberg, 'Can Patents Deter Innovation? The Anti-commons in Biomedical Research', *Science*, 280 (1998), 698–701.

Herold, Eve, *Stem Cell Wars: Inside Stories from the Frontlines* (New York: Palgrave Macmillan, 2006).

Holbrook, David, 'Medical Ethics and the Potentialities of the Living Being', *British Medicine Journal (Clinical Research Edition)*, 291 (1985), 1117–19.

Holbrook, David (ed.), *What is it to be Human? New Perspectives in Philosophy* (Aldershot: Gower Publishing, 1990).

Holderin, Fiedrich, *Patmos in Poems and Fragments*, quoted in Martin Heidegger, *Basic Writings*, ed. by David Farrell Krell (London: Routledge, 1978).

Hollick, Ann L., 'US Oceans Policy: The Truman Proclamations', *Virginia Journal of International Law*, 17:1 (1976), 23–55.

Holmila, Erkki, 'Common Heritage of Mankind in the Law of the Sea', in *Acta Societatis Martensis*, 1 (2005), 187–205.

Hopkin, Michael, 'Britain Gets Hybrid Embryo Go-Ahead', *Nature News* (5 September 2007/doi:10.1038/news070903-12). <http://www.nature.com/news/2007/070903/f ull/news070903-12.html> [accessed on 20 January 2008]

Humber, James M. and Robert F. Almeder (eds.), *Human Cloning* (Totwa: Humania Press, 1998).

Huxley, Aldous, *Brave New World* (London: Flamingo, 1994).

Institut Curie, 'Opposition Procedure with the European Patent Office', quoted in Matthew Rimmer, *Intellectual Property and Biotechnology: Biological Inventions* (Cheltenham: Edward Elgar publishing, 2008). <http://www.curie.net/actualities/myriad/declaration_e.htm> [accessed on 10 August 2008]

The Institutes of Justinian, trans. by John Thomas Abdy and Bryan Walker (Cambridge: Cambridge University Press, 1876). <http://www.archive.org/details/institutesofjust00abdyuoft> [accessed on 11 April 2004]

Interim Report on the United Nations and the Issue of Deep Ocean Resources, by United States. Congress. House. Committee on Foreign Affairs. Subcommittee on International Organizations, 90th Congress, First Session, 7 December 1967.

Irving,Dianne N., *Can Either Scientific Facts or 'Personhood' be Mediated?* <http://www.lifeissues.net/writers/irv_13persomediated.html> [accessed on 19 October 2004]

- - - *Philosophical and Scientific Analysis of the Nature of the Early Human Embryo.* <http://www.lifeissues.net/writers/irv/irv_36whatisbioethics12.html> [accessed on 23 November 2004]

Jensen, Kyle and Fiona Murray, 'Intellectual Property Landscape of the Human Genome', *Science*, 310 (2005), 239–40.

Jonas, Hans, *The Imperative of Responsibility: In Search of an Ethics for the Technological Age* (Chicago: University of Chicago Press, 1984).

- - - *Lasst uns einen Menschen klonieren*, quoted in Jurgen Habermas, *The Future of Human Nature* (Cambridge: Polity Press, 2003).

- - - *Memoirs*, ed. by Christian Wiese and trans. by Krishna Winston (Waltham, MA,: Brandeis University Press, 2008).

- - - *The Phenomenon of Life: Toward a Philosophical Biology* (Illinois: Northwestern University Press, 2001).

- - - *Philosophical Essays: From Ancient Creed to Technological Man* (Chicago: University of Chicago Press, 1974).

- - - 'Wissenschaft as Personal Experience', *Hastings Center Report*, 32:4 (2002), 27–35.

Joynor, Christopher C., *International Law in the 21st Century: Rules for Global Governance* (Lanham, MD: Rowman and Littlefield, 2005).

- - - 'Legal Implications of the Concept of the Common Heritage of Mankind', *International and Comparative Law Quarterly*, 35 (1986), 190–99.

Kameri-Mbote, Patricia, The Use of the Public Trust Doctrine in Law, Environment and Development Journal, 3:2 (2007). <http://www.lead-journal.org/content/0719 5.pdf> [accessed on 5 July 2008]

Kass, Leon R., Life, Liberty and the Defence of Dignity: The Challenge for Bioethics (San Francisco: Encounter Books, 2002).

- - - Toward a More Natural Science: Biology and Human Affairs (New York: The Free Press, 1988).

- - - 'Wisdom of Repugnance' in The Ethics of Human Cloning, ed. by Leon R. Kass and James Q. Wilson (Washington D.C.:AEI Press, 1998).

Kass, Leon R. and James Q. Wilson, The Ethics of Human Cloning (Washington D.C.: AEI Press, 1998).

Kevles, Daniel J., A History of Patenting Life in the United States with Comparative Attention to Europe and Canada: A Report to the European Group on Ethics in Science and Technologies (Luxembourg: Office for Official Publications of the European Communities, 2002).

Kirgis, F.L., 'Standing Challenge Human Endeavours that Could Change the Climate', American Journal of International Law, 84:2 (1990), 525–30.

Kiss, Alexander, 'The Common Heritage of Mankind: Utopia or Reality?', in Law of the Sea, ed. by Hugo Caminos (Aldershot, Hants: Ashgate/Dartmouth, 2001).

Kkorobkin, Russell, Stem Cell Century: Law and policy for a Breakthrough Technology (New Haven: Yale University Press, 2007).

Knoppers, Bartha Maria, 'Genetic Benefit Sharing', Science, 290:6 (2000), 49.

- - - 'The Human Genome: Individual Property or Common Heritage', in The Human Genome, co-ord. by Jean-Francois Mattei (Strasbourg: Council of Europe Publishing, 2006).

Knoppers, B., M. Hirtle and K. Glass, 'Commercialization of Genetic Research and Public Policy', Science, 286 (1999), 2277–78.

Koo, Dae Hwan, 'Effective Protection of DNA Sequences and Gene Innovations', in IIP Bulletin (2007). <http://www.iip.or.jp/e/summary/pdf/detail2006/e18_17.pdf> [accessed on 23 May 2008]

Krauss, Lawrence, 'The Physics of Star Trek' (London: Flamingo, 1997).

Lebacqz, Karen, 'Who "Owns" Cells and Tissues?', Health Care Analysis, 9:3 (2001), 356–68.

Ledeberg, J., 'Experimental Genetics and Human Evolution', The American Naturalist, 100:915 (1966), 519–31.

Lee, R.W., The Elements of Roman Law, 4th ed. (London: Sweet & Maxwell, 2007).

Lenk, Christian, Nils Hoppe and Roberto Andorno, Ethics and Law of Intellectual Property: Current Problems in Politics, Science and Technology (Aldershot: Ashgate Publishing Company, 2007).

Lenzerini, Federico, 'Biotechnology, Human Dignity and the Human Genome', in *Biotechnology and International Law*, ed. by Francesco Francioni and Tullio Scovazzi (Oxford: Hart Publishing, 2006).

Leveque, Francois and Yann Meniere, 'Patents and Innovation: Friends or Foes?', *Berkeley Center for Law and Technology*, 28 (2007).

Lewis, C.S., *The Abolition of Man* (New York: HarperCollins Publishers, 2001).

Li, Yuwen, *Transfer of Technology for Deep Sea-Bed Mining: The 1982 Law of the Sea Convention and Beyond* (Dordrecht: Martinus Nijhoff Publishers, 1994).

Logue, John J. (ed.), *The Fate of the Oceans* (Pennsylvania: Villanova University Press, 1972).

Lustig, B. Andrew, 'Natural Law, Property and Justice: The General Justification of Property', in *Thomas Aquinas*, ed. by John Inglis (Aldershot: Ashgate, 2006).

Mann Borgese, Elizabeth (ed.), *Pacem in Maribus* (New York: Doddy, Mead & Co., 1972).

Marcel, Gabriel, *Man Against Mass Society*, trans. by G.S. Fraser (Chicago: Gateway, 1952).

Mauron, Alex, 'Is the Genome the Secular Equivalent of the Soul?', *Science*, 291 (2001), 831–32.

McKibben, Bill, *Enough: Staying Human in an Engineered Age* (New York: Henry Holt and Company, 2003).

Merlo, Serano, 'The Meaning of Genome in Living beings: A Biophilosophical Approach', in *Human Genome, Human Person and the Society of the Future*, ed. by J. de Dios Vial Correa and E. Sgreccia (Vatican City: Libreria Editrice Vaticana, 1999).

Mitchell, Mark T., *Michael Polanyi* (Delaware: ISI Books, 2006).

Moore, Keith I., *The Developing Human: Clinically Oriented Embryology*, 3rd edn. (Philadelphia: WB Saunders Company, 1982).

Mossinghoff, Gerald J., 'The Evolution of Gene Patents Viewed from the United States Patent Office', in *Perspectives on Properties of the Human Genome Project*, ed. by F. Scott Kieff (Amsterdam: Elsevier Academic Press, 2003).

Murdoch Iris, *Sovereignty of Good* (London: Routledge, 2001).

Murray, Fiona, 'The Stem-Cell Market—Patents and the Pursuit of Scientific Progress', *The New England Journal of Medicine*, 356 (2007), 2341–43.

Murray, Michael H., *The Thought of Teilhard de Chardin* (New York: Seabury Press, 1966).

Nasif, Abdullah Omar, 'The Muslim Declaration of Nature', *Environmental Policy and Law* 17:1 (1987), 47.

Newman, Stuart, *The Role of Genetic Reductionism in Biocolonialism, quoted in Bill Mckibben, Enough: Staying Human in an Engineered Age* (New York: Henry Holt & Company, 2003).

Nordquist, Myron H., *United Nations Convention on the Law of the Sea 1982: A Commentary* (Dordrecht: Martinus Nijhoff Publishers, 1985).

Nuffield Council of Bioethics, *The Ethics of Patenting DNA: A Discussion Paper* (London: Nuffield Council on Bioethics, 2002).

O'Brien, Mahon, 'Commentary on Heidegger's "The Question Concerning Technology", in IWM Junior Visiting Fellows' Conferences, Vol. XVI/I, 2004.

Ossorio, Pilar, 'Common Heritage Arguments and the Patenting of DNA', in *Perspectives on Gene Patenting: Religion, Science and Industry in Dialogue*, ed. by A.R. Chapman (Washington D.C.: American Association for the Advancement of Science, 1988).

- - - 'The Human Genome as Common Heritage: Common Sense or Legal', *The Journal of Law, Medicine and Ethics of the American Society of Law, Medicine and Ethics*, 35:3 (2007), 425–39.

Pardo, Arvid, Address by Arvid Pardo to the 22nd Session of the General Assembly of the United Nations (1967), Official Records of the General Assembly, Twenty-Second Session, Agenda Item 92, Document A/6695.

- - - *The Common Heritage of Mankind: Selected Papers on Oceans and World Order 1967–1974* (Malta: Malta University Press 1975).

- - - 'First Statement to the First Committee of the General Assembly November 1, 1967', in *The Common Heritage of Mankind: Selected Papers on Oceans and World Order 1967–1974* (Malta: Malta University Press, 1975).

- - - 'The Law of the Sea: Its Past and Its Future', *Oregon Law Review*, 63:1 (1984), 7–17.

- - - Note Verbale to the Secretary-General, 22nd Sess., Annex, Mem., UN Doc. A/6695 (17 August 1967) (Request for the Inclusion of a Supplementary Item in the Agenda of the Twenty-Second Session).

- - - *'An Opportunity Lost'*, quoted in Kemal Baslar, *The Concept of Common Heritage of Mankind in International Law* (The Hague: Martinus Nijhoff Publishers, 1998).

Pardo, Arvid and Elizabeth Mann Borgese, *The New International Economic Order and the Law of the Sea: A Projection*, IOI Occasional Papers No. 4 (Malta: International Ocean Institute, 1975).

Pattison, George, *The Later Heidegger* (London: Routledge, 2000).

Peterson, Susan, The Common Heritage of Mankind?, *Environment*, 22:1 (1980), 6–11.

Plomer, Aurora, and others, Stem Cell Patents: European Patent Law and Ethics, European Commission (28 July 2006). <http://www.nottingham.ac.uk/law/StemCell-Project/project.reports.htm> [accessed on 12 June 2007]

Polanyi, Michael, *Knowing and Being* (London: Routledge & Kegan, 1969).

- - - 'Life Transcending Physics and Chemistry', *Chemical and Engineering News*, 45 (1967), 54–66.

- - - *Personal Knowledge: Towards a Post-Critical Philosophy* (London: Routledge, 2002).

- - - 'The Republic of Science: Its Political and Economic Theory', *Minerva* I (1962) 54–74.

- - - *The Tacit Dimension* (New York: Doubleday & Company, 1967).

Polanyi, Michael and Harry Prosch, *Meaning* (Chicago: The University of Chicago Press,1975).

Polt, Richard, *Heidegger* (London: Routledge, 2003).

President's Council on Bioethics, Alternative Sources of Human Pluripotent Stem Cells: A White Paper (Washington D.C.: May 2005).

President Lyndon Johnson's address, 'Remarks at the Commissioning of the Research Ship Oceanographer', delivered at the commissioning of the vessel, U.S. NOAA Oceanographer, on 13 July 1966.

Prows, Peter S., *Tough Love: The Dramatic Birth and Looming Demise of UNCLOS*. New York University Public Law and Legal Theory Working Papers, Paper 30 (2006). <http://lsr.nellco.org/nyu/plltwp/papers/30> [accessed on 15 June 2008]

Rae, Scott B. and Paul M. Cox, *Bioethics: A Christian Approach in a Pluralistic Age* (Michigan: William B. Eerdmans Publishing Company, 1999).

Ramsey, Paul, *Fabricated Man: The Ethics of Genetic Control* (New Haven: Yale University Press, 1970).

Reed, Esther D., 'Property Rights, Genes, and Common Good', *Journal of Religious Ethics*, 34:1 (2006), 41–67.

Regalado, Antonio, 'The Great Gene Grab', *Technology Review* (September/October 2000), 49–50.

Reichman, J.H., 'Saving the Patent Law from Itself: Informal Remarks Concerning the Systemic Problems Afflicting Developed Intellectual Property Regimes', in *Perspectives on Properties of the Human Genome Project*, ed. by F. Scott Kieff (Amsterdam: Elsevier Academic Press, 2003).

Reichman, J.H. and Paul F. Uhlir, Promoting Public Good Uses of Scientific Data: A Contractually Reconstructed Commons for Science and Innovation (working paper). <http://www.law.duke.edu/pd/papers/reichmananduhlir.pdf> [accessed on 10 March 2008]

Reimer, Tanya, *New Property and Global Governance: The Common Heritage of Mankind* (submitted by Tanya Reimer on April 24, 2007 to Dr. O'Brien in partial completion of Global Governance). <tanya.peatt.net/published/property_global_gov_chh.pdf> [accessed on 15 May 2007]

Reisman, Michael W., 'The Problem of Sovereignty and Human Rights in Contemporary International Law', *American Journal of International Law*, 84 (1990), 866–76.

Resnik, David B., 'A Biotechnology Patent Pool: An Idea Whose Time Has Come?', *The Journal of Philosophy, Science and Law*, 3 (2003). <http://www6.miami.edu/ethics/jpsl/archives/papers/biotechPatent.html> [accessed on 5 February 2005]

- - - 'DNA Patents and Human Dignity', *Journal of Law, Medicine and Ethics*, 29:2 (2001), 152–65.

- - - 'The Human Genome: Common Resource but not Common Heritage', in *Ethics for Life Scientists,* ed. by Michiel Korthals and Robert J. Borges (Dordrecht: Springer, 2004).

- - - *Owning the Genome: A Moral Analysis of DNA Patenting* (New York: State University of New York Press, 2004).

'Revised Preliminary Draft of a Universal Declaration on the Human Genome and Human Rights (20 December 1996)' in *Birth of the Universal Declaration of the Human Genome and Human Rights* (Paris: UNESCO, 1999).

Rifkin, Jeremy, *The Biotech Century: How Genetic Commerce will Change the World* (London; Phoenix, 1998).

Rimmer, Matthew, 'The Attack of the Clones: Patent Law and Stem Cell Research', *Journal of Law and Medicine,* 10:4 (2003), 448–507.

- - - *Intellectual Property and Biotechnology: Biological Inventions* (Cheltenham: Edward Elgar Publishing, 2008).

Roberts, Leslie R., R. John Davenport, Elizabeth Pennisi and Eliot Marshall, 'A History of the Human Genome Project', *Science*, 291 (2001), 1145–434.

Ronald, Duncan and Weston-Smith Miranda, *The Encyclopaedia of Ignorance: Everything You Ever Wanted To Know about the Unknown* (New York: Pocket Books, 1978).

Ross, Sir David, *Aristotle* (London: Routledge, 1996).

Rossi, Christopher R., *Equity and International Law? A Legal Realist Approach to the Process of International Decision Making*, quoted in Kemal Baslar, *The Concept of the Common Heritage of Mankind in International Law* (The Hague: Martinus Nijhoff Publishers, 1998).

Ryuichi, Ida, 'Human Genome as Common Heritage of Mankind—with a Proposal', *Bioethics in Asia*, 1.8 (1997). <http://www.eubios.info/ASIAE/BIAE59.htm> [accessed on 28 January 2008]

Sass, Hans-Martin, 'Why Protect the Human Genome', *Journal of Medicine and Philosophy*, 23:3 (1998), 227–33.

Schakelford, Scott J., 'The Tragedy of the Common Heritage of Mankind', *Stanford Environmental Law Journal* (Stanford Public Law Working Paper No. 1407332), 27 (2008).

Schrodinger, Erwin, *What is Life?* (Cambridge: Cambridge University Press, 2007).

Scovazzi, Tullio, The Concept of Common Heritage of Mankind and the Resources of the Seabed beyond the Limits of National Jurisdiction. http://www.iadb.o rg/.../Seminario_AUSPINTAL_2006_04_Scovazzi.pdf [accessed on 20 April 2007]

Seifert, J., 'Respect for Nature and Responsibility of the Person', in *Human Genome, Human Person and the Society of the Future*, ed. by J. de Dios Vial Crrea and E. Sgreccia (Vatican City: Libreria Editrice Vaticana, 1999).

Sevilla C. and others, The Impact of Gene Patents on the Cost-Effective Delivery of Care: The Case of BRCA1 Testing', quoted in Matthew Rimmer, Intellectual Property and Biotechnology: Biological Inventions (Cheltenham: Edward Elgar publishing, 2008).

Singh, N., 'Right to Environment and Sustainable Development as a Principle of International Law', *Studia Diplomatica* 41:1 (1988), 45–61.

Song, Robert, *Human Genetics* (Cleveland: The Pilgrim Press, 2002).

Sterckx, Sigfrid, 'Lack of Access to Essential Drugs: A Story of Continuing Global Failure, with Particular Attention to the Role of Patents', in *Ethics, and Intellectual Property: Current Problems in Politics, Science and Technology*, ed. by Christian Lenk, Nils Hoppe and Roberto Andorno (Aldershot: Ashgate Publishing, 2007).

Sterckx, Sigrid and Julian Cockbain, 'Patenting Human Embryonic Stem Cells', *PropEur* 3 (Winter 2006), Supplement. <http://www.propeur.bham.ac.uk/Newsletter% 20Vol%203%20Supplement.pdf> [accessed on 10 June 2008]

Strauss, Joseph, 'Product Patents on Human DNA Sequences', in *Perspectives on Properties of the Human Genome Project* (Amsterdam: Elsevier Academic Press, 2003).

Tatoud, Roger, Genes and Ownership; A Scientific Approach. <http://www.openDemocracy.net> [accessed on 10 January 2005]

Taylor, Charles, *The Ethics of Authenticity* (Cambridge M.A.: Harvard University Press, 1991).

- - - *The Explanation of Behaviour* (London: Routledge & Kegan Paul, 1980).

- - - *Sources of the Self: The Making of the Modern Identity* (Cambridge: Cambridge University Press, 2006).

Thomson, J.A. and others, 'Embryonic Stem Cell Lines Derived from Human Blastocysts', *Science* 282 (6 November 1998), 1145–47.

Thumm, Nikolaus, 'Patents for Genetic Inventions: A Tool to Promote Technological Advance or a Limitation for Upstream Inventions?', *Technovation* 25 (2005), 1410–17.

Tomuschat, Christian, Obligations Arising for States Without or Against Their Will, quoted in Peter S. Prows , Tough Love: The Dramatic Birth and Looming Demise of UNCLOS Property Law, New York University Public Law and Legal Theory Working Papers, Paper 30 (2006). <http://ssrn.com/abstract=918458> [accessed 15 June 2008]

Triggs, Gillian D. (ed), *The Antarctic Treaty Regime* (Cambridge: Cambridge University Press, 1987).

UN Sub-Commission on the Promotion and Protection of Human Rights, *Specific Human Issues: Working Paper on Universal Declaration on the Human Genome and Human Rights*, submitted by Antoanella-Iulia Motoc, 15 August 2002, E/CN.4/Sub.2/2002/37. <http://www.unhcr.ch/Huridocda/Huridoca.nsf/0/91ea34c 7ea607bb4c1256c1a0058857c/$FILE/GO215047.doc> [accessed on 10 May 2007]

UNESCO, *Birth of the Universal Declaration on the Human Genome and Human Rights* (Paris: UNESCO, 1999).

Virt, Prof. Gunther, 'Dissident Opinion', in *Opinion on the Ethical Aspects of Patenting Inventions Involving Human Stem Cells*, by European Group on Ethics, in Science and New Technologies to the European Commission, Opinion Number 16, 7 May 2002.

Wade, Nicholas, *The Quest for the $1,000 Human Genome,* quoted in Ronald M. Green, *Babies by Design: The Ethics of Genetic Choice* (New Haven: Yale University Press, 2007).

Watson, James D., DNA: *The Secret of Life* (New York: Alfred A. Knopf, 2003).

- - - *The Double Helix: A Personal Account of the Discovery of the Structure of DNA* (London: Weidenfield & Nicolson, 1968).

- - - *The Molecular Biology of the Gene* (New York: W.A. Benjamin, 1965).

Werpehowski, William and Stephen D. Crocco (eds.), *The Essential Paul Ramsey: A Collection* (New Haven: Yale University Press, 1994).

White, Lynn, 'The Historical Roots of our Ecological Crisis', *Science*, 155 (1967), 1203–07.

White, M.V., 'The Common Heritage of Mankind Principle: An Assessment', *Case Western Reserve Journal of International Law*, 1982 14 (1982), 509–42.

Whiteman, Marjorie M., Digest *of International Law*, 15 vols (Washington D.C.:U.S. Government Printing Office, 1963–1973), II (1963), 1030–1232.

Wilberg, Peter, Human Ontology or Human Genomics: Heidegger's Health Warning to Humanity. <http://www.meaningofdepression.com/human%20Ontology.ppt> [accessed 20 January 2009]

Wildiers, N.M., *Teilhard de Chardin* (London: William Collins Sons & Co., 1969).

Wolin, Richard, *Heidegger's Children* (Princetown: Princetown University Press, 2001).

Worrell, Richard and Michael C. Appleby, 'Stewardship of Natural Resources: Definition, Ethical and Practical Aspects', *Journal of Agricultural and Environmental Ethics*, 12 (2000), 263–77.

Zaner, Richard M., 'Surprise! You're Just Like Me! : Reflections on Cloning, Eugenics, and Other Utopias', in *Human Cloning*, ed. by James M. Humber and Robert F. Almeder (New Jersey: Humana Press, 1998).

Zimmerman, Michael E., 'Beyond "Humanism": Heidegger's Understanding of Technology', in *Heidegger the Man and the Thinker*, ed. by Thomas Sheehan (Chicago: Precedent Publishing, 1981).

Zitzelsberger, Hilde. M., 'Concerning Technology: Thinking with Heidegger', *Nursing Philosophy*, 5:3 (2004), 242–50.